GET FIT, LEAN

AND KEEP YOUR DAY JOB

A Transformation Guide For Any Body

J. D. Griffin

Edited by Steve Welch

Cover photo by Rich Frye

Illustrations by Maurice Laflamme III

TRX and Suspension Training are registered trademarks of Fitness Anywhere LLC

Precor and AMT are registered trademarks of Precor Incorporated

Hammer Strength is a registered trademark of Brunswick Corporation

Visit the author's website at getfitlean.com

Visit the author's facebook page at https://www.facebook.com/GetFitLeanAndKeepYourDayJob

Published by Griffin Books

Copyright © 2014 by J. D. Griffin

All rights reserved.

ISBN: 0990565610

ISBN 13: 9780990565611

Disclaimer

For Faris and Zianah.

Please eat your vegetables.

Love,

Dad

Standing in a checkout line you notice the cover model on a fitness magazine. You think to yourself, "I'd love to look like that, but I'd have to hire a nutritionist and workout six hours a day."

Not so! As a working father of two, calling me busy is an understatement. I transformed my flabby middle-aged body into the body of a chiseled men's physique competitor. The only thing standing in the way of your transformation is you.

A full-time fitness career is not a requirement. Armed with the right nutrition, cardio and resistance training plans, you can transform yourself in much less time than you think.

This book is a guide for anybody and any body. It's a no nonsense program that will transform your body in twelve weeks and maintain the new you for life.

You will shed fat, build lean muscle and learn how to maintain a constant energy level all day.

Commit for twelve weeks, follow my program and I will deliver you a new you.

Prologue

My Inspiration

In the spring of 2009 I moved from Houston, Texas to the San Francisco Bay area in northern California. I'd recently gone through a difficult period in my life and had gained a lot of weight. Disgusted with how I looked and felt, I decided to make a change. I entered a twelve-week body transformation challenge and lost thirty pounds while gaining lean muscle. Just after completing the contest in June of 2009, I posted my before and after pictures on my Facebook page.

A lot of friends saw those pictures and asked me how I did it. They also asked me to write down my meal diary and training plan. So I created a simple three-page document and sent it to a handful of friends. Apart from a few detailed questions, I didn't hear much back. Three months later while visiting Houston, I stopped by the office of an ex-colleague to say hello and grab lunch. I bumped into a second old friend, Jade. What surprised me about our chance meeting is that Jade had completely transformed his physique - he looked great!

Jade and I had worked together the previous year while I was living in Houston. The best description of him then would have been a typical skinny fat man. Jade had a pretty good-sized potbelly and no muscle tone on his thin arms. He was in his mid-thirties, a father of two, and he hadn't participated in sports or stepped foot in a gym since high school.

Seeing Jade for the first time since I'd left Houston six months earlier, I was shocked. Jade looked like a new man. He had completely transformed his body composition. He'd lost all of his belly fat and now had a chiseled chest and powerful arms. In stunned disbelief I said, "You look great, what have you been doing?" Jade replied, "I followed your 'Get Fit, Lean' program." I couldn't believe it. Another friend had printed a copy and given it to Jade, and he then followed it. Standing before me was a prime example of how my Get Fit, Lean program could work for the average person. Jade had grown tired of what he'd let himself become. After he'd seen my before and after pictures on Facebook, he dedicated himself to follow my program for twelve weeks. I had no idea he'd ever even seen my program, let alone followed it.

Jade told me that he felt great, his self-esteem had never been higher and he couldn't remember ever having so much energy. His wife loved the way he looked now, and she had just started following my program as well. Knowing I'd helped an old friend improve his quality of life was a great feeling. It made me realize I had something special with this program.

Since then, I've helped a lot of other people achieve great results. Men and women, young and old, overweight and thin, I've been able to help a lot of people who've wanted to help themselves. My Get Fit, Lean program has expanded far beyond that initial 3-page summary, and the book you are now reading is a comprehensive guide to transforming yourself. It includes all the detail needed for anyone to succeed. Everything you need to know plus many helpful hints is what follows in this book. I hope you enjoy it - and better yet, I hope you follow it.

Sincerely,

JD

Contents

Eat Clean, Train Hard, and Sleep Well. Repeat.

Like you, I'm a busy person with many different interests. I'm an involved father of two overscheduled kids and I work a full-time job. Most nights I go to bed feeling like there is never enough time in the day to squeeze in all the things I'd like to do, let alone *need* to do. The fact is, most of us are very busy. That's life. We can't change the fact that there seems to always be more to do than there are hours in a day. We can, however, learn to prioritize better, manage our time better, and make the most out of our precious little free time. Commit just a small fraction of your day to getting fit and lean and you can succeed in completely transforming your body.

Would you like to lose your belly fat, flab, fat rolls, and build lean muscle? Would you like to get fit but you think you'd have to spend hours a day in the gym? You *can* get fit and it doesn't require hours a day. Consistency is the key. Not having enough time is not a valid excuse. If you really want to make a change, you can and will find the time. Do you think it's too complicated or unrealistic? It's not. Getting fit and lean is simple and it's a realistic goal for anybody. I got rid of my belly fat and built lean muscle. There's no good reason why you can't make the same transformation.

My goal in writing this book is to provide a simple, practical, and comprehensive guide that anybody can use to shed fat, gain lean muscle, and build a fit, lean body. This is the Get Fit, Lean program. And it WILL change your life if you follow it.

The last five years of my life have been truly transformational. At 49 years old, I now look and feel better than ever. Friends, family and even complete strangers often ask me how I'm able to stay as fit as I do, especially at my age. It's not complicated. I honestly believe that anybody can do it. Therefore, I'm sharing my program with everybody that truly wants to make a change but just doesn't know where to begin or what to do. Maybe you, like I had at one point, resigned yourself to living the rest of your life as just another ordinary out-of-shape person already on the back nine of life. You don't have to go out this way. It's never too late to decide you are ready to make a change and transform your body. Picking up this book is the first step. Let's move on and keep it rolling right now.

Armed with the Get Fit, Lean program, you too can transform your body from out of shape and flabby to fit, lean, and younger looking. I know this because I did it – and you can too. I'm going to share with you everything you need to know about how to get there. Out of shape and fat or fit and lean? It's your choice. It's time to Get Fit, Lean.

Dear Friend:
This Is Your Reality Check

If you need to get in shape, lose some weight, and improve your health you are not alone. The majority of Americans, and for that matter most people living all over the globe from the rich western world to the underdeveloped third world, are overweight.[1] Unfortunately, the trend is continuing in the wrong direction as the percentage of obese people around the globe continues to grow. Obesity is even on the rise in poor countries. The spread of readily available fast foods, processed foods, manufactured fats and other junk foods is largely responsible. A greater percentage of the world's population is obese than ever before in human history.[2] Obesity is truly a growing global epidemic.

Obesity is linked to several very destructive and preventable diseases and conditions. These health problems include but are not limited to type II diabetes, heart disease, high blood pressure, dementia, back pain, and joint problems just to name a few. Author Dr. Robert Lustig groups all of these obesity-linked diseases into what he calls Metabolic Syndrome.[3]

Why be part of the trend? Just because most people are killing themselves eating these ever-more-convenient food-like products doesn't mean you have to follow the herd. Instead of following the lemmings over the cliff, you can walk your own path and choose the healthy fitness lifestyle.

No Punches Pulled

This book is intentionally written in the friendly tone of an honest conversation. Consider me your fit friend that you've come to for help. You're tired of the way your body looks and you've decided enough is enough. You want to make a change. We meet to talk where I promise you I'm going to give it to you straight and be completely honest. Sometimes it might be that I'm too honest. Brutally honest. But that's how I am. It's like Ferris Bueller said in his namesake movie, "You don't respect someone who's kissing your ass." You won't respect what I'm telling you if I'm not honest. Therefore, I'm not going to pull any punches or sugar-coat anything. I promise you no BS. Are you ready? Here goes.

You look the way you do because you eat a lot of garbage. You make excuses and have convinced yourself that you don't have the time to exercise or go to a gym. Or that you'll start tomorrow. Or next week. Or next year. Well, friend, the time is today. Make exercise a priority and you will make the time. You can find the time to go to the gym. You kid yourself into thinking you don't actually eat THAT bad -- but you're wrong. You eat just about anything and everything that tastes good with no regard for nutritional value. You consider most all food equal, whatever it may be. If it tastes good, you eat it. You, like most people, are driven by short-term satisfaction with little to no regard for long-term health consequences.

You may think that your lack of fitness and/or excess weight is too far gone. You might also think that you've reached the point of no return. Neither is the case. There's no such thing as too far gone. It's never too late to make a change. You may have even convinced yourself that you look "ok." Stop kidding yourself, you don't. Like many people, your self-perception is probably very distorted. For men, this is the reality of our oversized fragile male egos. A fundamental difference in the sexes is how men and women perceive themselves. Ladies, you're already one step ahead of us guys. Women are better able recognize the problem.

For example, a woman with a nice body will look at herself in the mirror and see her flaws. She'll obsess over every tiny imperfection. She'll think she looks too fat or too thin or too something. This is just how some women are wired. Whereas when a completely ordinary average man looks at himself in the mirror, he sees something very different from reality. He sucks in his gut and puffs up his chest then thinks, "I'm just a couple pounds away from posing for the cover of a fitness magazine." Wrong! Try twenty, thirty, maybe many more pounds away and seriously deficient on lean muscle. It's the male ego at work. Most guys have a greatly exaggerated perception of themselves. Women on the other hand are too hard on themselves, obsessing over the smallest imperfections. This is just how we semi-advanced apes are wired. For men and women both, you've come to the right person for help. I'm going to help you make a permanent change. Follow my Get Fit, Lean program and in 12 weeks you'll look and feel like a whole new person.

Workout Fails

I'm going to point out a few more brutally honest observations on what a lot of people are doing wrong. I'm not trying to be overly negative here, but I am willing to bet that the majority of the people reading this book are making or have made some of the mistakes I'm about to point out. These are common "Workout Fails" and if any of them apply to you, then we're already on the road to improving your fitness regimen.

Workout Fail #1: The Fitness Club Socialite

Some people, more often guys but also some of you gals, already spend a lot of time at the gym "working out" with your buddies. The truth is it's more of a social scene than an actual workout for too many people. I see too many guys who spend most of their time in the gym standing around talking about sports, television shows, and sex. They occasionally try to impress each other with how much they can bench press or do a few sets of curls.

Gentlemen, maybe no one's ever been honest enough to tell you this so let me be the first. You only impress each other. Not a single woman anywhere cares that you can bench press 315 pounds for reps. You are able to bench press a lot of mass because you are a lot of mass. You're carrying a lot of excess body mass, that is. Here is the hard cold reality my friend. No woman is ever going to ask you how much you bench press because they couldn't care less. Ladies don't find the big round smooth look attractive either. The gym goon look just isn't sexy to women. What gals do like is chiseled abs, defined arms, rock solid chest and shoulders. The lean muscular athletic beach body look is what they find attractive. You'd be hard pressed to find any women who disagree. So spend less time and energy talking and trying to impress the people around you, and focus on the task at hand: a short, intense workout that is far more effective in burning fat and building muscle. I'll outline this process in the following chapters.

Workout Fail #2: The Cardio Junkies

Many women, but occasionally men too, mistake skinny and thin with fit. They spend all their time in the gym doing some sort of cardio exercise, sometimes hours on end. They never touch a weight or do any kind of resistance training and then starve themselves. Their nutrition plan consists of eating very little of anything. Skinny is not sexy, thin is not sexy - Fit and Lean is sexy.

Workout Fail #2.5: The Starvation "Diet" (usually done in conjunction with the Cardio Junkie)

Eating just enough to survive is not a healthy "diet" plan much less a sustainable lifestyle – but it's one of the most common fails. Not eating enough food can deplete muscle mass and bone density, and is extremely unhealthy. Such a diet ends up cannibalizing the body's muscle tissue, the very engine in the body that burns the most fat. Excessive cardio and poor nutrition is counterproductive. Neither food nor calories are the problem. The wrong foods and wrong calories are the problem. Calories are not the enemy; a healthy body requires fuel in the form of calories. But it needs quality fuel. Your body needs calories from the right food sources. Balancing a good nutrition plan and resistance training with the proper amount of cardio will make anyone look and feel so much better. The chapters on nutrition will explain in detail and give you the facts and guidance you need to supercharge your body and turn it into a lean fat-burning machine.

Ok, you probably get the idea. I could write a whole book on workout fails, but I won't. Now that I've focused on some of the negative, let's start focusing on the positive. Because my Get Fit, Lean program will make a profoundly positive impact on your life.

The Positives:
Positive #1: Getting Fit and Lean Feels Good

Living the Get Fit, Lean lifestyle is rewarding both physically and psychologically. Feeling good is as big a part of it as looking good. So let's talk about looking and feeling good. Through hard work and dedication following the Get Fit, Lean program, I've now got a standout physique. I'm one of those people that walk into a room and often get double takes. Sometimes I find myself in a conversation with a woman and catch her checking out my chest or arms. Admittedly, it's both very flattering and a heck of a lot of fun. It's a great feeling. Who doesn't want to feel good about themselves? Some people confuse that with being egotistical. It's not about ego. The fact is, getting noticed gives you tremendous self-confidence and boosts your self-esteem.

I didn't always feel this way. I remember feeling terrible when I was over-weight, lacking in both self-esteem and self-confidence. I was embarrassed to take my shirt off at the beach or even tuck my shirt in - instead always trying to figure out how to hide my shape. My body was inflated, and my self-esteem was deflated. It's true that you've got to like yourself before other people will like you, and that people will see you the way you see yourself. So I'm here to help you get fit and lean and like yourself more. Boosting your self-image and self-esteem will make people see you differently. And nobody should be ashamed of feeling good about themselves.

Would you like to rebuild your self-confidence and self-esteem? To never again worry that you can't wear certain clothes? You can be the one who can get away with wearing anything and look good. The person who walks confidently into a company meeting not afraid to stand up in front of a group and speak when asked. Be the person who doesn't think twice about wearing a bathing suit on vacation or to the pool with your kids. Maybe even the person that turns heads just walking down the street. Follow my program and you can be that person.

Positive #2: Longevity

We all want to live long lives and we're all familiar with the notion of survival of the fittest. A great deal of scientific evidence strongly suggests that physically fit humans will walk this earth a far greater length of time than overweight unhealthy specimens – and they'll enjoy the time they're here a lot more, too. Multiple studies have shown that physically fit people have a far lower risk of dying from any cause compared to the least fit.[4] It's true. Fit people live longer than overweight people. And when you're fit and healthy, those extra years are a heck of a lot more enjoyable.

You've got to want to do it for yourself first, but another great motivator is to get fit for the people in your life who love and care about you. Do it for yourself, but also do it for your friends and family. You can be sure that your children, grandchildren and all your family would like to see you stick around above ground as long as possible.

Positive #3: Improved Physiology

Our bodies are continuously in the process of rebuilding themselves.[5] Our blood-rich muscle tissue has particularly strong rejuvenating properties, which makes a twelve-week transformation possible for anybody. Think of it in these terms. Three months from now your muscle cells will have rebuilt themselves anyway.[6] Stay on the same old path you're on now and all you'll get is further deterioration.

Instead, commit to my Get Fit, Lean program and rebuild your muscle tissue with a stronger, healthier upgrade. No matter what your present condition, age or genetic makeup, with some dedication, determination and a little hard work you too can transform yourself into a new you.

"Obsessed is a word the lazy use to describe the dedicated"

- Russell Warren

My Fitness Journey

My first ever encounter with serious fitness enthusiasts was with the hardcore bodybuilding crowd I met my freshman year in college. By chance, I lived in the same dorm as my school's football team and became friends with a few of the players. Like me, these guys were eighteen years old but unlike me they had some serious muscle development. They got loads of attention from the girls and a lot of respect from the guys. I started working out and getting some not-so-good advice from them. As a naïve college freshman I was easily persuaded to try steroids.

I ended up experimenting on and off with different steroids throughout my four years of college, putting on around forty extra pounds of very round muscle-like mass. By the way, my modest gains were small compared to what some guys achieved by stacking multiple drugs. Looking back on this time in my life I now know my friends and I were just dumb kids. We knew next to nothing about good nutrition or proper training. We ate as much of whatever we could get our hands and often trained the same muscles, usually chest and arms (the mirror muscles), three times a week. Our primary objective was to "get as big as a house." I did. I became a very round, smooth, not very athletic looking house.

After graduating college in the spring of 1987 I moved my big round muscles to Chicago. I was flat broke and heavily in debt so I took two jobs that first summer. One of those jobs was as a bouncer in a popular nightclub on Division Street and the other a lifeguard at an upscale high-rise building on the Gold Coast. I didn't have the time or the money for a gym membership, and certainly least of all the funds to support my four-year steroid habit. By the end of the summer, just a few months later, the nightclub management was wondering why the 215-pound scary looking meathead bouncer they'd hired shrunk down to a 175-pound normal looking skinny kid. Thankfully they liked me and allowed me to move from bouncer to bartender where I excelled at the craft, but that is a whole other story.

Drug free and workout free for just 3 months, it was as if I'd never touched a weight or stepped foot in a gym in my life. The lesson here is an obvious one, I hope. Gains from steroids are temporary. As soon as you get off the "juice", or "gear" as it's more commonly called now, the effects begin to wear off fast. Most of what you get taking steroids is water retention, acne, aggression and who knows what kind of long term internal damage. So my advice is, don't touch steroids. The muscle gains are only temporary and the side effects aren't worth the health risks.

Soon after, I found a full-time job and then had the time to work out on a regular basis once again. As far as building my physique was concerned, I was starting from scratch all over again. The positive lesson I learned from my gym experience in college was how to train hard with focus and intensity. That's a lesson I've been putting to good use ever since. I also promised myself this time around I'd do it naturally with no performance enhancing drugs of any kind. My mission became to prove it could be done drug free. I'm proud to say that the muscle development I now have is one hundred percent the result of hard work and good nutrition.

Average Genes

Like most of the population, the genetic make-up I inherited falls right in the middle of a normal distribution. Physically, I'm a pretty average ordinary guy. My parents blessed me with an average build. There are no "Arnolds" or RGIIIs in my family tree. Had I picked a different set of parents, *i.e.*, won the genetic lottery, I'd likely not written this book, as I'd probably have cashed in on a lucrative NFL contract or I'd have become a famous Olympic athlete.

As it turns out I was dealt a different hand, average genes. But like other things, being average is not a hall pass to let yourself get or stay out of shape. Anyone can get fit and lean. Like many people, I once blamed my inability to make gains and get in better shape on poor genetics, but I now realize that it was just an excuse. One thing that I've learned over the years as I've gotten more and more into the fitness lifestyle and the physique competition world is that in the long run, good nutrition and hard work trumps everything. Through good nutrition, consistent hard work and dedication, you can achieve greatness. You too can transform your ordinary body into a lean beautiful physique.

My Transformation

The subprime housing meltdown and subsequent banking crisis indirectly led me down the path I'm on now. In the fall of 2008 I was laid off from the bank I worked for. A short time after, a routine medical exam turned into two anxiety-filled months of visits to specialists along with some invasive tests. To top it all off, my marriage was falling apart. Depressed, I thought the end was near so I sought comfort by gorging on my favorite decadent foods and copious amounts of red wine. I gained an obscene amount of weight, quickly becoming physically grotesque while my self-esteem sank to all-time lows.

Fortunately, the medical scares turned out to be nothing more than false alarms. I found a new job and worked out an amicable separation with my then wife. Meanwhile, I'd gained over thirty pounds of flab. I looked and felt worse than I ever had in my life. Fed up with what I'd let myself become, I decided to do something about it.

At the age of 43 I entered a twelve-week body transformation contest. The contest essay that I submitted to the judges is included in the back of this book (Appendix A). I didn't win the transformation contest, but I was very proud of the results I achieved. I lost over thirty pounds of fat and have kept it off. I never imagined then that entering a body transformation contest would be so truly life changing or that the experience would put me on the path I'm on now.

Five years later, I look and feel better than ever. Like anything else in life, the more you practice something the better you become. It's no different with nutrition and exercise. As you learn how your body responds, you'll continue to become more and more dialed in.

A Lifestyle Choice

What sometimes felt like real work or an inconvenience five years ago has now become my lifestyle - and it's surprisingly easy to maintain. I'm hooked on feeling good. In fact, I love training and look forward to my time working out every day. I strongly believe that exercise clears the mind and cleanses the body. Cardio training purges the toxins from my body. The resistance-training pump gives me a confidence boost and positive energy that I carry with me all day long. Exercise doesn't feel like a chore. I can't imagine not doing some sort of exercise every day. I think that like most things you do in life, once you commit to the lifestyle and just start doing it, it quickly becomes part of your day-to-day routine.

I've also learned, admittedly out of necessity, to be extremely time efficient when it comes to working out. After thirty plus years of integrating some kind of workout routine into my daily schedule, I've learned to minimize the time required and maximize the results. I'm sharing all the time saving efficiency tips I've learned over the years with you in this book.

From the plastic sand-filled weight set my brother and I worked out with in our parent's basement as teenagers to the hard-core collegiate weight rooms to the Masters 45+ Men's Physique competitions of recent years, fitness has been a big part of my life for a long time. I've learned volumes along the way about what works and what doesn't work. It's all in my program and I share it all.

You Already Know Me

I'm the guy at your office, the neighbor down the street or the old friend who you consider the obsessed workout junkie. You tease me at office parties when I'm the only one turning down cake and ice cream. I'm the guy who orders the grilled chicken breast salad instead of a sandwich and chips when we go out for lunch. I'm also the guy who orders a green vegetable and skips the pasta dish with my dinner. When you see me out for a run or bike ride at the crack of dawn, you think to yourself, *what's wrong with this guy?* You wonder how I find the time to work out consistently six to seven days a week. You probably even joke about how boring I must be. I don't mind. In fact, I hope my lifestyle inspires others to try harder to look after their fitness, stay strong, eat healthy, and live more productive lives. After all, there are much worse addictions in life than being a fitness junkie.

I Also Know You

But no matter what you may say in jest, we both know the truth. You'd love to change your body composition. Few people wouldn't. That's why losing weight and getting in shape are two of the most common New Year's resolutions every single year. When you get out of the shower and look at yourself in the mirror do you like what you see? Be honest. You're probably disappointed in what you've let yourself become. Let's face it; a pouch of a belly, sagging rear end, and little to no muscle tone are not exactly attractive features. You'd love to look better but you don't know where to start or don't think you have the time. The idea of building a fit, lean body seems too daunting, overwhelming or simply unrealistic. Maybe you believe that weight gain is part of the aging process. You accept your sagging belly, flabby bottom and deteriorating muscle tone as just a fact of life. You've come to believe that it's just part of getting old. Well, I'm here to tell you – and prove to you – that it doesn't have to be.

You may still be young, in your twenties or thirties. Maybe you were allowed to eat all the candy and fast food you wanted as a child. You're young but have the body of an out of shape overweight middle-aged person. There's a good chance you're well on your way to obesity, heart disease, type II diabetes and for women, osteoporosis. Maybe you think that you're just too far gone. You believe it's not possible to change so you've just given up and don't even bother trying to eat healthy or even consider exercising. One of the first things you have to do is stop thinking like that. You CAN turn it all around. You're never too far gone.

How can you turn it around? It's simple: make your fitness a priority and you'll find that you do have the time and you can find the energy. All you have to do is make the commitment to change. My Get Fit, Lean program provides the instructions for transforming your body into a lean machine bursting with self-esteem. A fit lean body lives within your body. The fit lean you is just hidden away under something else and together we're going to get rid of that something else.

The 16th century Renaissance artist Michelangelo thought of sculpting as freeing a beautiful figure trapped inside stone. In his mind's eye the art of sculpting meant removing the excess stone to free what was already there. He thought of his works of sculpture as freeing beautiful trapped human forms with his chisel. What you may have trouble seeing right now is your lean body trapped inside a lot of excess body mass. The lean version of you is in there. You've just got to set it free. My program is your chisel. If you commit to following my program, you'll be taking the first step in setting free your trapped lean body.

Why Listen to Me?

I did it. You should listen to me because *I did it*. I transformed myself from a potbellied, over-weight 43-year-old middle-aged man into a fit lean physique competitor. It's much more than just getting ripped in 12 weeks for a contest. Most importantly, it's about maintaining your health and fitness for life. Look at my before and after pictures to see what you can achieve in just 12 weeks and then look at me now, five years later at age 49. I look and feel better now than I ever have.

Learn from a guy who's done it. I'll share everything with you. Over the years I've been my own guinea pig and learned much by trial and error. The experiment was on me. My kitchen and the many gyms I've belonged to were my laboratories. I've been continually working on this experiment for the last 30+ years with some significant results. I've tried everything from steroids in college to various fad "diets" over the last three decades. I've tried power lifting, bodybuilding routines, extreme cardio routines and popular diet routines that have come in and out of fashion. I've also trained with a long list of athletes and countless experienced personal trainers. My point is that I know what works and what doesn't. Because of all those years of experimentation, the most important thing of all is that NOW I know how to get results. I've taken a huge catalog of information and distilled it down into the Get Fit, Lean program. Everything that worked for me can and should work for anybody who's willing to commit. I want to help anyone who truly wants to make a change.

Enough of my sermon. Let's get started!

Chapter 1

"Everything should be made as simple as possible, but not simpler."

- Albert Einstein

Program Basics

Can't wait to begin to get fit and lean? If you want to get started today, right now, you can. Please do read every chapter of this book, but there's no reason why you have to wait until you've finished them all to get started. There are a lot of simple enough lifestyle changes you can make right now that will have an immediate impact on the way you look and feel. There's no reason to put off what you can begin right now.

My Get Fit, Lean program is divided into three functional sections: (1) Nutrition plan, (2) Cardiovascular Exercise plan and (3) Resistance Training plan. Nutrition is everything you eat and drink. Cardio is exercise that gets your heart rate up and makes you sweat. Synonymous terms for resistance training are weight training and strength training. I'm going to go over the basics of each of these in this chapter, but as you can see I devote multiple chapters to each one later in the book. Think of this chapter as the CliffsNotes for the whole book.

Basic #1: Nutrition

I made nutrition #1 because it is most important. If you don't fuel your body right, everything else will hardly even matter. Nutrition is 80% of getting fit and building lean muscle, not to mention maintaining good health for life. You can sweat buckets of perspiration doing hours of cardio and pump iron like an Olympian, but if you live on a high-calorie diet of junk food you'll likely not even put a dent in the problem. Good nutrition is fundamental to getting fit and lean. The food you eat fuels your brain and body, gives you energy for working out, aids recovery and provides the building blocks for lean muscle growth. From the perspective of nutrition, the most common way that we measure and compare all the food and drink we consume is by the number of calories they contain.

What Exactly Is a Calorie?

Trying to make sense of all the different dietary claims and popular diet tag lines concerning calories can be very confusing. You might hear one dietician say that a calorie is a calorie is a calorie. Then, you'll hear another nutritionist say that not all calories are created equally or that calories count or that calories *don't* count. Which is it? How do you make sense of all the hype and noise surrounding calories? I want to begin my nutrition discussion by defining the mysterious calorie.

Much like an ounce is a unit measure of mass, a calorie is a unit measure of energy. A calorie is the amount of energy required to raise the temperature of one kilogram of water by one degree Celsius. So, in fact, a calorie is a calorie.

An ounce of lead and an ounce of gold are two very different things yet both are still an ounce. The two metals have very different values. An ounce of lead is worth about $0.006 and an ounce of gold is worth about $1,300.00 because they have different properties.

In the context of nutrition, there are important differences between calories, depending on the food sources. Different food sources have different properties. The number of calories from two different food sources can be equal, yet have very different properties, and therefore have very different effects on your body. For example, 1 oz of cooked chicken breast is 28 calories, 1/4 oz of white sugar is 28 calories, and 1/3 oz of 100 proof vodka is also 28 calories. Eating the chicken breast helps repair muscle tissue, eating the sugar spikes your insulin release system and drinking the vodka has an entirely different effect. So although a calorie is a calorie, it makes a *HUGE* difference where those calories come from in terms of transforming your body. Eating the right number of calories is important, and eating calories from the right food sources is equally important. That's why I spend a lot of effort in this book discussing macronutrients and the differences between various types of foods.

What to Eat: Food and Macronutrients

The basics of good nutrition are pretty simple. Eat ***intact whole foods*** made up of lean proteins, healthy fats, and **un**processed carbohydrates in the form of fresh, mostly green vegetables, whole grains and limited fruits. Do not eat processed foods. Especially avoid refined carbohydrates. Refined carbohydrates are produced when whole plants are stripped of their fiber and nutrients leaving only highly digestible sugar or starch. The most common and problematic refined carbohydrates are sugar, typically made from the sugar cane plant, and flour, typically made from grains.

Keep meal planning simple. Try to include one fresh whole food item from each of the three macronutrient groups in each meal. The three macronutrients are proteins, fats and carbohydrates. If your macronutrient food sources are a variety of fresh whole foods, then your micronutrients like vitamins and minerals should be covered. Just to be sure, I do recommend that you take a high quality vitamin and mineral supplement, daily.

Sample menus are included in a later chapter but I love to talk about food – it's THAT important - so here are some good meal examples to start with. A typical breakfast could be scrambled egg whites, a sliced avocado, fresh salsa and whole grain bread or whole grain tortillas. Another breakfast choice could be whole grain oatmeal with a scoop of your favorite protein powder, a couple tablespoons of natural peanut butter, and topped with blueberries or strawberries. Lunch and dinner choices are also pretty easy. Grilled chicken breast, asparagus or spinach lightly sautéed in olive oil and a side of baked sweet potato is a great meal. Another lunch or dinner choice could be baked fish, whole grain brown rice and steamed broccoli, cauliflower or grilled asparagus.

Snacks

Always keep healthy in between meal snacks nearby. Don't put yourself in a situation that tests your will power over the call of the vending machine or the plate of homemade chocolate chip cookies in the break room that Betty Sue brought into work for the office to share. There are a lot of healthy snack options you can keep nearby for those moments when you've just got to eat something. I know. I've been there. Set yourself up to succeed by always having a healthy food alternative nearby.

One great midday snack option is unsalted almonds. They're not only a great source of healthy fat, they're also calorie dense, making them very filling. Just a handful can tide you over between meals. Bring an apple, banana, or some other piece of fruit to work for another healthy snack alternative (although I will discuss why you should limit your fruit intake later). Low glycemic fruits like cherries, blueberries, blackberries and strawberries are the best fruit choices but an apple or orange is still much better than a candy bar or bag of potato chips. If you've got access to an office refrigerator keep a container of low-fat cottage cheese or plain Greek yogurt, a great source of protein, hidden behind that waist expanding twelve-pack of cola you'll never touch. Even better, buy a mini-fridge and keep it under your desk at work so your healthy snacks are always close by. Natural peanut butter (with no sugar added) is also a great snack option. Just a couple tablespoons can tide you over until your next meal. Don't wait until you're hungry to think about these snacks, plan ahead. Keep the healthy snacks nearby to ensure you don't falter in a moment of weakness. The smell of those cookies can be awfully powerful, so always have a healthy alternative on hand. Failing to plan is planning to fail.

Basic #2: Cardio/Work Up a Sweat

The cardio aspect of the Get Fit, Lean program is also pretty simple. Move your body, get your heart rate up, and sweat. We are designed to move, not to sit behind a desk and surf the Internet all day, although it does seem that some folks are paid to do just that. Take inventory of how you spend your time every day and challenge yourself to find an hour to workout. Surf the Internet less, play fewer video games or tear yourself away from the TV in the evening and get your body moving. A good cardio burn is about getting your heart rate up, not so much what exercise you choose. This may seem simple, and it is. Good fitness doesn't have to be overly complex, especially if you're not particularly active now.

If you prefer the controlled climate of an indoor gym then join a spin, step aerobics, circuit training or a Zumba class. You may, however, prefer to go it alone rather than do classes with a bunch of other people. If so, hop on a stationary bike, elliptical machine, stair machine or a treadmill. If you're the outdoors or nature loving type, then run, jog, mountain bike or road bike. Swim, box, grapple, jump rope, skinny ski, whatever gets your heart rate up. The point is to move your body and work your cardiovascular system. Even if all you do is a fast walk around the block, congratulations - you're lapping all the people sitting at home on their couch. That's it. Get active and do SOMETHING cardio-focused for 30-40 minutes five to six times a week (or more if you can).

Basic #3: Resistance/Weight/Strength Training

The basics of resistance training are also pretty simple. Train with intensity and train to failure. It's the last rep that counts. I'll show you how to optimize your time spent resistance training and get the most out of every workout's exercise, set, and rep. The weight training routines in my Get Fit, Lean program are time efficient. You do what it takes to stimulate your body's adaptive growth response then you move on, nothing more. Focus.

If you've never touched a barbell or stepped foot in a gym in your life, don't worry. The chapters that follow discuss how to get started and safely train with free weights, weight machines and resistance exercises that only require your own body weight. In no time at all you'll be pushing yourself beyond what you thought you'd ever be capable of. Don't worry that you'll have to use heavy weights because you won't - it's not about how much weight you're using. It's about tapping your body's hard-wired adaptive response by training to failure. Stimulating muscle hypertrophy (growth) is what matters. Training to failure stimulates your natural growth response. Combine that with the right nutrition plan and fit, lean muscle will follow.

Your starting point also makes no difference. Whether you're overweight (even obese) and need to lose weight or seriously skinny and want to build lean muscle, it doesn't matter. Either way, the Get Fit, Lean program is for you. I will address the transformation strategies for each body type, although other than the nutrition plan they're not a whole lot different from one another. When done together, the basic principles will work for anyone, plain and simple.

Program Summary

Everything you need to know to succeed will be covered in detail in the following chapters. You can get started now. You don't have to wait. Eat whole intact foods from the three macronutrient groups, proteins, fats and carbohydrates. Do some cardio, get your heart rate up and sweat. Resistance train with focus and intensity and push each set to failure. These are the three components of my program. It's really and truly that simple. All three will be covered in detail in the following chapters.

My Get Fit, Lean program is intentionally easy to follow, time efficient and practical. Remember, my primary goal in writing this book is to provide a simple comprehensive guide that anybody can use to shed fat, get lean and build a good looking body.

Chapter 2

"A journey of a thousand miles begins with a single step."

- Lao-tzu

It's a Lifestyle Not a Diet

To begin with, I don't like to use the word "diet." We're going to strike the word diet from our vocabulary. This is not a "diet" book nor am I advocating in any way that you "go on a diet." The word diet has an implied meaning contrary to what you're trying to achieve. There are much more accurate words that refer to how you choose to fuel your body. Instead, refer to what you choose to eat as your meal plan, eating plan, nutrition plan or simply your *nutrition*. As I noted previously, Basic #1 is nutrition. This is not a diet.

A diet implies an interim deviation from your "normal" eating habits. The term diet implies something temporary, as in "I'll go on a diet" then once it's over I'll go off it. Diet also implies a short-term fix, designed to achieve a desired weight loss goal. The problem with diets is that they are typically abandoned after some fixed period of time, and then the dieter returns to their previous "normal" eating habits and gets fat again. A temporary fix is not your goal. **Good nutrition is a lifestyle, not a diet.**

Additionally, most "diets" are doomed to failure in the long run because they are not designed with long-term health in mind. They are neither sincere lifestyle changes nor are they genuine healthy long-term nutrition plans. The reality is that most diets are little more than clever marketing ploys designed to sell books or videos or food products by promoting a so-called "new" and never-before-heard-of diet plan. Sure, some of them can help you temporarily lose weight. Atkins, South Beach, The Grapefruit Diet, The Zone Diet; the list of popular fad diets is never-ending. The problem is few of them offer a practical, healthy and sustainable nutrition plan for life. Even the bits of good information are hard to find buried in unnecessarily complicated material and too often interwoven with unhealthy or unsustainable advice.

I'll cut through the information overload and give it to you straight in simple, easy to understand and follow practical terms. My nutrition plan outlines what you need to eat and not eat in order to shed fat and build lean muscle. It also outlines sensible nutrition guidelines to follow after reaching your goals in order to avoid rebounding. It will eliminate the kind of yo-yo effect between eating clean and binging that often comes after "diets". Get Fit, Lean is a healthy practical nutrition plan for life. The most important step you can take right now is to commit yourself and be disciplined.

A Lifestyle, Not a Diet

A "lifestyle," unlike a "diet," is a long-term plan. A lifestyle is something you adopt permanently. It's a game plan for healthy living that you follow for as long as your heart's still ticking and you're walking around above ground. Nine out of ten health experts surveyed agree that your above ground time can be significantly lengthened through good nutrition and exercise. Think of your nutrition plan as part of your personal rules for living, your personal policy or parameters. This is pretty simple yet important. The Get Fit, Lean nutrition plan is the framework for building the new you.

Everything that you put in your body either hurts you or helps you. From an extreme point of view you can look at food as just another drug. Everything you eat or drink is then either poison or medicine. Junk food can be just as destructive as and just as addictive and poisonous to your body as illicit drugs. Some people struggle with junk food addictions much like other people struggle with drugs, alcohol, and other chemical addictions. Recreational drugs, including junk food can be extremely destructive. Doing any of these drugs is something that falls outside of your personal health and nutrition boundaries. Think of drinking a cola loaded with 42 grams of high fructose corn syrup or gorging yourself on cake and cookies as no different than snorting, smoking or injecting some destructive recreational drug. Is it really so different? Say no to the poisons and stick with the medicines. Get off the refined carbohydrate fix and instead eat clean. Eating clean means eating fresh intact whole foods and not eating any overly processed garbage. Stick to your nutrition plan, do your cardio training and do your resistance training. Stick to the program and you will be successful.

Smart Food Choices

We're faced with countless food choices all day every day. Throughout the course of any given day we are bombarded with bad food choice opportunities. They seem never-ending and come at us in an infinite number of tempting forms. There are a few choices that you absolutely need to be aware of, so that you can make the right choices about what to eat – and what NOT to eat.

Never Eat Fast Food Again

This may seem like a no-brainer, but the fact is, millions of people eat fast food on a regular basis. While driving on a long road trip, hungry and thirsty, the all-too-familiar glistening golden arches appear on the horizon. Or maybe you're running late after work or you've got little time for lunch, and need to find something fast and convenient, and lo and behold, there's a fast food joint right in front of you. So you think, well, this one time is ok... WRONG. Don't give in to that temptation. Sometimes it's sheer willpower that gets you through, so be strong. Don't swap your long-term health and fitness goals for short-term gratification.

What the fast food chains lack in quality ingredients and good nutrition they make up for in taste. I'll be the first to admit it; a big juicy cheeseburger, fries and cola taste really good. They've got the taste formula down, but remember how awful you're certain to feel minutes later. It's no coincidence that you'll feel like crap either, because fast food burgers usually contain actual crap. That's right, mass market "ground beef" used in fast food is washed out with ammonia to kill the *E. coli* bacteria.[7] It then has to be artificially flavored in order to make it taste and smell like meat again. Don't put that in your body. Ever.

Fast foods and other junk foods are cheap, convenient, and they usually do taste good as well. They should taste good. Corporate fast food giants spend millions on research and development formulating great tasting products with little consideration for the nutritional value or the source of the ingredients. The many food-like products they sell are often loaded with hormones, antibiotics, artificial additives, chemical preservatives or other not-so-natural ingredients.[8] Nutritional content is the least of their concerns. Corporate food giants have stockholders to keep happy. What do you think is more important to a publicly traded company, making their quarterly earnings targets or your long-term health and well-being? The fact that they're fattening up the masses with their food-like products is of little consequence to them. They're not interested in your long-term health. Therefore, you've got to look out for yourself and make informed intelligent food choices. Fast food should be completely off the list of anyone who is serious about their health and the health of their families. I'm pretty sure that if you eat fast food, your kids are eating it too. Do yourself and your family a favor and cross this junk off your food list forever.

After Work Social Hours

Another good choice opportunity occurs when the office party crowd tries to convince you to come along for happy hour. "Just one, we promise, we'll make it an early night," they plead. Yeah, right, does that ever happen? Once you've made the decision to get fit and have committed yourself to a new lifestyle then it's easy to say no to the bad choices. Are you really going to give in to peer pressure and derail your fitness plan just to feel like crap the next morning? This isn't high school my friend; who cares what the party people think? Be your own person, walk your own path and do what's right for you. Some things just don't fit in with your lifestyle. Let other people fund the ever-growing type 2 diabetes and heart disease medicine research industry. When you live the fitness lifestyle, excess food and drink is just no longer your cup of tea. But don't get me wrong, I'm not suggesting you can't go out or you can't be social. You can and you should, but you have to have some limits and make good choices.

The key to success is consistency. This means sticking with the program day to day, every day. Your transformation isn't going to happen overnight. It's a process. But if you stick to the program you'll start seeing and feeling results in a matter of days. Stick with the program for the entire 12 weeks and you'll see dramatic results. When you're invited out for "a couple of drinks," be very careful. Temper the "ok, just this once" response at least until you reach your fitness goal. When you do join friends in a social setting that involves alcohol and heaping plates of nachos, learn to order an iced tea, coffee or water and find something healthy to eat. If the people you're out with are true friends, they will support your lifestyle choices. You don't have to be a lemming. You have to be true to you, and you have to be strong.

Additional Benefits

In evolutionary terms, building and maintaining muscle is very expensive. Muscle is expensive because muscle requires additional energy both to build and to maintain. Building and maintaining muscle is costly in terms of calories required. Continual physical stress is also required in order to maintain muscle strength and size. Our bodies are in a constant state of adapting to our current environment. If the demands you put on your muscles are greater than their capacity, they will adapt by growing stronger and bigger. Conversely if the stress you put on your muscles is less than their capacity, they will adapt by shrinking.[9] This is simply the conservation of energy, an adaptive survival mechanism, playing out in real time.

Our bodies are highly efficient machines that have evolved to adapt to environmental stresses. If you're not using your muscles, then they are wasting expensive calories and become unnecessary to maintain. We're designed then to use it or lose it. However, this adaptive mechanism can actually suit us well. If you have access to adequate quantities of healthy foods (or better stated, as good calories) then you can build and maintain lean muscle mass. We've evolved to do so. Understanding our evolutionary design is important. To get a fit, lean body, you need to know that you have to put continual stress on your muscles just to maintain them. Our muscles are designed to grow or shrink depending on how we use them.

If you are a super user of modern convenience, you are directly contributing to your own physical deterioration. Let's say for example that you drive to work every day, park in a garage and take an elevator to your office. You then sit at your desk most of the day and the only work you do is typing on a keyboard. Someone else prepares most if not all of your meals. After work you go home, sit on a couch, watch TV, play video games, surf the Internet and read a book until you go to bed. You wake up and repeat the same rigorous routine day after day. If this is you, you're putting almost zero physical stress on your body. Your body will adapt by shrinking, causing you to lose both muscle and bone mass (osteoporosis). The Get Fit, Lean program will help you adapt and evolve too – from a sedentary lifestyle to an active one that will result in positive changes in your body – created by you through good nutrition and exercise.

Counteracting Osteoporosis

The stress of exercise not only benefits our muscles. The stress of exercise also benefits our skeletal system a great deal as well.[10] We did not evolve to drive cars everywhere, sit in chairs all day and stare at computer monitors. We are designed to move, putting physical stresses on our bodies. For the last several million years our ancestors had to work hard day-to-day just to survive. Getting their heart rates up and stressing their muscles was part of everyday life. It's unnatural to lead a sedentary existence. If no physical stress is put on our bodies then we will lose both muscle and bone mass. We effectively age faster than we have to. Part of the natural aging process is a gradual loss of muscle and bone mass, but do you really want to accelerate that? Wouldn't you rather slow down the process? You can.

Osteoporosis is a relative newcomer to the list of human debilitating diseases. Women are especially at risk. Like many other modern afflictions, osteoporosis is largely a result of our modern sedentary lifestyles and poor nutrition.[11] A good nutrition plan ensuring adequate vitamins and minerals, particularly calcium in this case, coupled with regular exercise (especially resistance training) is the best preventative plan to stave off osteoporosis. This is why I recommend that everyone should lift weights. This is especially true for women and it becomes more and more important as we age. Lifting weights or using weight-bearing resistance equipment puts stress on our bones and in turn they respond by retaining their strength and density.

Chapter 3

"You can't out train a bad diet."

- Unknown

Avoiding Processed Poisons

Enjoying delicious food is an important part of my life and it's probably an important part of yours. I love good food and I love to eat well. I really don't think I could live the fitness lifestyle if I wasn't able to enjoy eating great tasting foods. I've an appreciation for good food and love experiencing different foods from all the world's cultures. There are, however, some foods that are simply off limits. Delicious, healthy food choices abound, and there are certain "foods" you have to absolutely avoid.

Eating Fresh, Intact, Whole Foods

First, let's clearly define what real or whole foods actually are, because it's often not clear. Unfortunately, we are overwhelmed daily with an abundance of readily available "food-like" products masquerading as real food. Clever marketing firms design shiny packages, craft advertising campaigns, and write catchy jingles, all trying hard to persuade you to cram a lot of man-made food-like products into your mouth. What makes these engineered products especially difficult to avoid is that they usually taste pretty good. When loaded with enough sugar, salt and artificial flavors, it's possible to make almost any rubbish taste great. Here's the straight dope: these food-like products are not food. We modern humans are not designed to deal with consuming and digesting them nor are we able to extract much, if any, nutrition from them. We're designed to fuel our bodies with fresh intact whole foods, not food-like products packaged in a box or vacuum wrapped in plastic. The good news is that with a little effort and creativity, you can make fresh whole foods taste better than any manufactured food that's been engineered in some corporate R&D lab.

Whole Foods Versus Processed Foods

Whole foods are naturally occurring whole intact non-processed foods that provide real nutritional value. Technically, *food processing* is any deliberate change to a food before it's eaten. Freezing, drying and cooking are all forms of food processing that preserve nutritional value. Therefore, for the purpose of this discussion, the processed foods I'm referring to are foods whereby the processing has either destroyed, degraded or stripped the original whole food of most, if not all, of its nutritional value. The processing was done for reasons of shelf life and taste, with no regard for nutritional content.

Food products like white sugar and refined flour are made using a process that strips away, degrades or destroys the nutritional value of what was previously a whole food. For the purpose of this discussion, the most harmful processed foods I'm referring to are the refined carbohydrates white sugar, fructose and white flour. These processed foods that I'm advocating you stop consuming are foods whose nutritional value has been devalued or stripped away completely.

Getting fit and lean means you'll need to stop eating the nutritionally void processed foods, period. Refined carbohydrates have a great deal of energy value (calories) but little to no nutritional value. If the excess energy isn't burned imme-diately, our bodies will store it as fat. Refined carbohydrates, particularly refined sugars, are the primary culprits that cause weight gain and wreak havoc on the body's insulin release system.[12]

There is plenty of good news ahead in coming chapters but let's start by getting the bad news out of the way first. I say bad news only because if you're like me, a lover of life, you probably do indulge in decadent foods once in a while. Most of us love the taste of fresh pasta, warm bread made from refined flour, steamed white rice, cookies, cake, pie, maybe even doughnuts, and the list goes on. Therefore, I'm sorry to tell you that these foods made from refined carbohydrates are like a poison. They don't help you; instead they only hurt you. Start thinking of refined sugar and refined flour as addictive, dangerous and destructive recreational drugs. Like heroin, cocaine or any other illicit drug, refined carbohydrates have no place in your new healthy lifestyle. But don't worry, the good news is that there are plenty of delicious whole foods you can replace the nutrition-less processed foods with and continue to enjoy great tasting meals. I'm a bit of a "foodie." I love great food and I also love to cook. In a later chapter I'll talk about great tasting foods that you should be eating, but first let's continue talking about what is off limits. Remember, it's a lifestyle not a diet.

Clean Eating Rule #1: Eliminate Refined Carbohydrates

The primary objective of the Get Fit, Lean program is to both lose fat and build lean muscle. To do this, it's imperative to eat clean. Clean eating rule number one is this: you've got to cut out refined carbohydrates. Adopt a zero tolerance. Why? Because eating refined carbohydrates causes your insulin release system to spike and the insulin spike is the root cause of why we get fat (I'll explain this in more detail soon). So, consider processed foods, particularly refined carbohydrates, to be like heroin and consider yourself a recovering junkie. You've got to go cold turkey. Later on, after you've achieved your weight and body composition goals, you can very occasionally eat some processed carbohydrates as part of a "cheat meal." But for now, stick with the plan: none, nada, nil, zero.

If you follow Rule #1, you're 80% home. People who know me well joke that I'm the sugar Nazi. I consider white sugar and white flour to be pure evil. My belief is these refined poisons were created deep in the bowels of hell. While these (in the loosest sense of the term) "foods" may not actually originate from the underworld, they will certainly plump you up nicely and cause multiple health problems. For those of you whose goal is building layers of unsightly belly fat and developing chronic metabolic syndrome diseases including terminal heart disease and type II diabetes, keep stuffing yourself with processed carbohydrates. For everybody else, eliminate them; they are your number one nemesis.

Our Genetic Pre-Disposition to Store Fat

Right now you might be saying, "Hey, JD, what's so terribly wrong with refined carbohydrates? Why do I have to give them up entirely? Isn't that a little extreme?" Please allow me to explain. It has to do with our genetic and physiologic pre-disposition to store energy reserves as fat. We are first and foremost hard-wired for survival. When presented with the opportunity, our bodies are well adapted to store as much excess energy as possible. However, we are not well adapted to deal with processed carbohydrates. Humans are biologically designed to eat intact whole foods, not processed foods, particularly refined carbohydrates. We have no mechanism to efficiently deal with the latter.

In working out a solution to any problem, I believe you should first try to understand the root of the problem. Let's begin by taking a look at the course of human evolution as it relates to food. Understanding that we are hardwired for survival and how our biochemistry deals with food will help you stay on your good nutrition plan. It will also make your fat loss and lean muscle goals easier to achieve.

For the first several million years or so of human history there were no fast food drive-thru windows, mega grocery stores or big box retail chains. Sprawling store shelves stocked with an endless number of processed foods didn't exist. Our cavemen ancestors had to work hard, sometimes for days, to find food and when they did, the feast was on. Take Lucy for example, the now world famous Australopithecus from the Ethiopian desert. Lucy lived 3.2 million years ago and is the grandmother of us all.[13] Truth be told, Lucy was in fact an indulgent party girl at heart. When Lucy and her clan made a big kill or stumbled upon a ripe fruit tree, they gorged themselves with as much food as they could. This made perfect survival sense. They didn't know where their next meal was coming from or when that might be. They fattened themselves up in times of plenty in order to make it through the lean times. After millions of years of this behavior our bodies are well adapted to dealing with occasional bountiful food finds between long periods of scarcity.

We are hard-wired, programmed and designed to store excess energy as fat reserves at every opportunity.[14] So the problem with eating refined carbohydrates is that doing so leads your body to believe that every meal is just such an opportunity. We are not designed to deal well with the blood sugar overload and subsequent insulin spike that comes from eating refined carbohydrates.[15] Rather, we are perfectly designed to eat intact whole foods, period.

The Critical Role of the Hormone Insulin

This next process concerning our insulin release system is something I absolutely need you to read carefully and understand. This is the cornerstone to the Get Fit, Lean program as it relates to fat loss. Here it is:

Intact whole foods are the optimal fuel for our beautifully designed machines. The carbohydrates (sugars and starches) in whole foods such as fruits, vegetables, and whole grains are bound in fiber, and therefore they are digested slowly. Naturally occurring sugar bound in fiber does not cause the insulin spike that our bodies are ill equipped to deal with.[16] You may be wondering what I'm talking about in terms of this insulin spike, so let me explain fully.

As any carbohydrate is digested, our blood glucose (blood sugar) levels rise. Now, because our bodies always want to stay in a state of balance, those rising blood sugar levels then trigger our pancreas to release insulin. The hormone insulin triggers our liver to convert the blood glucose in our blood stream into glycogen. Glycogen is a molecular structure that binds strands of glucose together as a means of storing energy. Glycogen is stored primarily in our liver, skeletal muscle, and fat cells. Therefore, the key to losing fat and staying lean is to eliminate insulin spikes. When we eat a reasonable quantity of intact whole food carbohydrates, our blood sugar is slowly elevated, and then insulin is in turn released in small quantities, and does not trigger an insulin spike. This is how our insulin release system is supposed to function.

In sharp contrast to our reaction to eating whole foods, our insulin release and glycogen storage system is poorly adapted to deal with refined sugars and flours that have unfortunately become a staple of our modern world's food supply. We haven't evolved to deal with the blood sugar spike caused by eating processed carbohydrates, especially sugar. Eating refined carbohydrates triggers a very different insulin response. When we eat refined carbohydrates, they cause our blood sugar level to rapidly spike to unnaturally high levels. This is turn causes our pancreas to flood our bloodstream with insulin. That spike in insulin then causes our body to go into hyper-absorption and store the excess blood sugar as fat. Our bodies store all that they're able to store and then some. Doing this repeatedly will cause your body to store fat in large quantities rather quickly. And, not only can this repetitive process make us fat, it can eventually lead to insulin resistance and diabetes among other metabolic syndrome related diseases. This is why rates of obesity and diabetes have surged in the US and anywhere that people have adopted the Western diet high in sugar, flour, and other refined processed carbohydrates. Dr. Robert Lustig, author of *Fat Chance*, groups all of the obesity linked diseases such as type II diabetes, heart disease, high blood pressure, and dementia into one category: Metabolic Syndrome. So now you can understand why I am constantly preaching about avoiding processed carbohydrates, such as sugar and flour. Consuming them makes you fat and leads to a long list of health problems. Period.

History and Refined Carbohydrates

As I've previously mentioned, for the first several million years of human evolution processed foods like white sugar and white flour didn't exist. Consequently, when you walk past the natural history museum's caveman exhibit you might think to yourself, "That guy is a little hairy but he sure does have great looking abs." Well, there's a reason for that. Refined carbohydrates were only developed a few hundred years ago and only became readily available post World

War II. The problem has even accelerated since the 1970s with the invention of deriving fructose from corn. It's all happened rather fast and we humans haven't had time to adapt. If he were alive today, Charles Darwin would be the first to tell you that evolution occurs slowly over the course of many generations.

The most common processed carbohydrates are refined sugar and white flour. From your body's point of view, white sugar and white flour aren't very different. Our biological response is about the same. Consuming either one of these causes a blood sugar spike, insulin flood and hyper-drive fat storage. Refined sugar primarily comes from sugar cane, palm sugar, sugar beet, sucrose, lactose, and fructose (often derived from corn). Sugar's function in food products is to deliver a sweet taste sensation and very temporary energy boost. Refined flour and sugar have a high energy content but zero nutritional value. Yet they have become a major staple in our diets. How did this happen? Well, you can blame our ancestors.

Biscuits on the Wagon Train

Refined flour is basically a product of the industrial revolution. In the good ol' days, transporting perishable food items over great distances and long routes presented a big problem. Breads and other foods made from milled flour had a very limited shelf life.[17] These foods wouldn't stay good packed in covered wagons for the extended journey across the Great Plains. There was a serious need for non-perishable flour. The grain milling process exposed the fatty acid of the germ to oxygen, which dramatically limited its shelf life. This created a major problem because the exposed germ would quickly go rancid.[18] Therefore, removing the germ was deemed to be the solution to the spoiling problem. Without the germ, flour cannot become rancid – and so refined white flour was born.[19]

In the flour refining process, fiber and nutrients contained in the bran and the germ are removed and thrown away. What remains has virtually no nutritional value, only an energy value or calories. But refined flour is much less perishable and therefore traveled well. It became the perfect non-perishable processed food product for the covered wagon migration across the prairie. I doubt the first people who came up with the idea of refining sugar and flour would have ever guessed that just a few generations later their innovation would contribute to a global obesity epidemic. White sugar sweetens grandma's iced tea and refined flour helps make cookies chewy and taste good. But these processed carbohydrates wreak havoc on our body's insulin release system, which just happens to be our body's fat storage trigger.

Regulating the Insulin Response to Limit Fat Storage

The release of the hormone insulin is a natural mechanism that allows us to store energy for later use. When it's working properly, it allows us to function normally and healthily. What is most important is to regulate and control it. We can do this by consuming intact whole foods. The energy content of intact whole food is bound in fiber, and therefore slowly digested elevating our blood sugar level gradually. When we eat whole intact foods our insulin release is slow and steady. This is how we're actually designed to store energy from the food we eat.

Hard-wired for survival, our pre-programmed survival adaptation to store fat is perpetually switched on and it has no off switch. This was a great survival mechanism when the wildebeest herd moved on for the winter and our ancestors were stuck boiling roots and eating tree bark until spring. The problem in our modern world is that all the cheap processed foods and refined carbohydrates are readily available at every fast food drive through, quickie mart and grocery store you come across – and as a result too many people eat them constantly, with every meal and almost every snack. Their bodies are in a constant state of insulin spikes and fat storage mode. So there you have it. The key is to eat the right foods and regulate that insulin response in your body. Once you understand this, it makes getting fit and lean a lot easier.

Stay the Course and Eat Clean

As you embrace the Get Fit, Lean Program, it's crucial that you maintain good discipline. If you do fall off the wagon and pig out on some kind of processed carbohydrates just once a day or even just once a week, you risk minimizing or even totally negating your fat loss. So I'm going to keep telling you, don't do it, don't trigger the insulin spike and hyper fat storage mode. You can store a surprising amount of glycogen as fat in just one meal so it's very important not to allow this to happen. Be strong. Commit yourself to your fat loss goal and your new healthy lifestyle choice.

Good nutrition means eating the right intact whole foods in reasonable quantities. Doing this triggers a healthy slow steady release of insulin. It's important that you do this because putting an end to the insulin spikes will allow your desired fat loss to occur. The most effective fat burn is slow and steady. Anytime you screw up in a moment of weakness and chow down on that deep dish pizza, cheeseburger and fries, ice cream, candy bar or piece of pie, you trigger an insulin spike. You're then signaling your body to store as much glycogen as possible – and guess what it's stored as: FAT. Even if it's just a few times a week, you're negating the slow steady fat burn you're trying to achieve the rest of the time. Do you really want to undo a whole week of sweat equity for a few minutes of short-term satisfaction? Fit and lean feels better than any junk food tastes.

The Steady Energy Benefit

Five years ago when I did my 12-week body transformation contest I experienced an unexpected benefit: a steady, sustained energy level all day. Once I began eating clean, I had a constant steady energy level throughout the day. When you give up refined carbohydrates and adopt a healthy nutrition plan, the insulin spikes, sugar highs and inevitable energy crashes disappear. This is one of the greatest benefits of a healthy lifestyle, particularly the nutrition plan.

I don't get tired mid-day. I don't experience the energy highs and lows that I once did. There are other factors I'll talk about later on but cutting out the refined carbohydrates is the single biggest variable in the consistent energy equation. My constant steady energy level helps me to perform better in all things I do. I stay better focused and am more productive both at work and in my personal life. I love it. I'm truly able to get the most out of my day every day. And you will too, by following the plan.

Obesity Epidemic

Unfortunately, most of the world's population is either unaware, just doesn't care, or simply eats whatever they're spoon-fed. These folks are generously contributing to the worldwide obesity epidemic. Take a look at this exploding worldwide epidemic. It began in the mid-19th century then picked up speed just after World War II and it's continuing to grow today. As developing nations adopt our modern western diets of convenience and processed foods the obesity epidemic is exploding on a global scale. The United States and Germany are in a dead heat for the top spot in the world's fattest population contest but China, India, Mexico and other developing nations aren't far behind.

So what's fueling the obesity epidemic? As mentioned earlier the main reason is very simple: processed carbohydrates are cheap and have become the primary food for a large part of the world's population. Evolution has designed us to not just store a little fat but as much fat as we can.

Pre-Programmed to Store Fat

As you know by now, our bodies are hard-wired for survival and have evolved to store energy reserves as fat. Our biological reaction to whatever food we eat is the release of insulin and absorption of blood sugar. Whether it's a tasty wooly mammoth burger or a delicious sun ripened peach, our bodies turn whatever we've eaten into blood sugar or blood glucose. Insulin is then released into the blood stream, which triggers an absorption response. Glycogen is then stored in our red blood cells, liver, skeletal muscle cells and fat cells. To make matters worse, we've also evolved to have a taste for and even crave energy-rich sugar. This is more of the ol' survival mechanism at work. We've evolved to like sweet tasting foods.

It's no coincidence that fruit ripens just before the onset of winter in the fall. There's a symbiotic relationship between plants and animals. Our ancestors added extra fat to their bodies by gorging themselves on sweet ripe fruit in the fall. Along with other animals, humans in turn spread the seeds helping the plant species survive. It's nature's way.

Until recent human history this pre-programmed disposition to store fat has served us well. Our ancestors were driven by hunger and a taste for sugar and salt. Storing fat is a great survival strategy. However, this mechanism has created a serious problem for modern humans. Eating processed foods presents many problems that we are simply not equipped to deal with. If you're a hunter/gatherer living on the African plains and have to survive for weeks between meals then storing fat may very well save your life. But unless you're training for a Japanese Sumo Wrestling Team, modern day humans do not require such an aggressive biological response for storing fat.

Bear with me please. My "processed foods and refined carbohydrates are poison" sermon is almost over. I realize I'm driving this point home pretty hard. One might even say ranting and raving a bit. Guilty. If the only thing you take away from my nutrition plan or from this entire book is just this one point then it's worth it. Breaking the processed carbohydrate habit and learning to regulate your insulin response could very well save your life. Stop eating refined carbohydrates! Do this alone and you'll be eighty percent home in terms of fat loss and long term health.

Pre-Digested Food

A not so pleasant way to think of eating processed carbohydrates is like this. When we eat refined carbs most of the digestive "work" has already been done for us. It's not far off from consuming pre-digested food. I'll stick with the example of ordinary white table sugar. Sugar, made up of sucrose and fructose, is the biggest culprit in the growing worldwide obesity epidemic.[20] What we humans are designed to consume is whole intact foods. The carbohydrates that occur in whole foods such as fruits, vegetables and grains is bound in fiber which requires our bodies to work in order to convert the food into blood sugar. The slow break down and conversion to blood glucose does not trigger an insulin spike. Conversely, when we eat a refined carbohydrate like table sugar our bodies have almost no work to do in the digestion process. Fructose (white table sugar is half fructose and half glucose) and high-fructose corn syrup are just a small bio-chemical step away from glycogen to begin with. They are therefore effortlessly converted to glycogen, responsible for triggering an insulin spike that in turn stores it as fat if not burned immediately.

Additionally, when you choose to eat processed carbohydrates instead of intact whole fruits and vegetables, you're missing out on the many benefits of fiber, which has been shown to help the colon and cleanse our digestive tract. I'm sure you've heard or seen the popular marketing term, "heart healthy." Foods such as avocados and whole grains are heart healthy, whereas refined carbohydrates are not. Our body's insulin release system reacts very differently when we eat fiber-dense intact whole foods. Instead of the overwhelming flood of insulin, a steady amount of insulin is slowly released. When we eat intact whole foods we avoid the otherwise unavoidable insulin spike and the inevitable energy roller coaster that follows.

Energy Highs and Lows

Let's talk a little more about energy levels. Everyone is likely all too familiar with the post meal sugar buzz and subsequent "food coma." Admittedly, the one occasion I allow myself to seriously overeat is Thanksgiving Dinner. I just refuse to give up this one annual indulgence. It's a tradition rich with fond childhood memories of turkey, stuffing, mashed potatoes, cranberries and gravy. Stretching out afterwards on a couch and slipping into a drooling food coma while watching a football game is of course unavoidable. I think one day a year falling horribly off the wagon isn't going to do any real long-term damage. The problem is there are people who treat every day as if it were Thanksgiving! This is why they get fat and lethargic and continue on the same cycle day in and day out. If this describes you, then it's time to break out of that vicious cycle, my friend.

I was once one of these people. My typical lunch was a big sandwich loaded with processed lunchmeat, pseudo-cheese food, and mayonnaise on white bread, a bag of chips and either a soda or a diet soda (it didn't matter really, because they're equally bad for you in many ways, and even elicit the same biological response). Chowing down on this popular lunch combination provided immediate gratification when I felt hungry. But what I was consuming was just a big load of refined processed carbs, salt, saturated fat, and all sorts of artificial preservatives and flavorings. Guess what happened next?

The struggle to remain conscious would begin shortly afterwards. My insulin release system spiked because we're poorly equipped to shove 2,000 calories of refined carbohydrates in our mouth, especially in one sitting. The result at first was a very brief sugar high followed by the inevitable energy "crash." Desperate to stay awake a short while later I'd stagger to the nearest vending machine to down another soda and/or cram a candy bar in my mouth, repeating this ugly cycle all day. I can tell you from firsthand experience that being trapped on this roller coaster is no fun. Get off the sugar roller coaster ride and make a change. Fat and trapped or fit and free; it's up to you to decide.

I remember living this way. It now seems like a distant past life. The post-lunch sugar buzz crash was so severe I literally couldn't keep my eyes open afterwards. God forbid I had to attend a meeting shortly after my mid-day processed carb load. I can even remember sitting around a conference table in a business meeting where I was supposed to be an active participant. The struggle not to nod off in front of everyone was overwhelming. My productivity, along with that of a lot of other folks in my office, went to zero for a couple hours immediately following lunch every day. Sound familiar? Sound inefficient? I can tell you that it's embarrassing, to say the least.

Avoid Calorie-laden Drinks

What we eat isn't the only source of refined carbohydrates. A major source of empty calories that many people aren't aware of – or that they simply underestimate – is the sugar in soft drinks, sports drinks, energy drinks, and other popular bottled beverages. They cause that same insulin and fat-storage response. Therefore, it's EXTREMELY important to avoid drinking your calories from sugar-loaded drinks! More sugar is consumed via soft drinks than any other delivery system.[21] Soda, cola, fountain drinks, soda-pop, whatever you want to call it depending on where you grew up, it's all loaded with sugar or high-fructose corn syrup. Sodas have a nutrient density of zero. Think of them, as the Center for Science in the Public Interest does, as liquid candy. [22] Therefore, don't touch another drop.

Before consuming any food or drink, you should always take the time to read the label first. Many so-called pre-workout drinks, recovery drinks and energy drinks are also loaded with sugar. A lot of people drink bottles of Gatorade or Monster Energy drink not realizing they're just drinking sugar-loaded water with a few vitamins, electrolytes and/or caffeine added in order to make it sound healthy or better than soda. It's not. The bottom line is, you have to read the label. If it's got added sugar, then don't touch it. Sugar = insulin spike = fat storage. Got it? I'll talk later about clean ways to get a caffeine jolt, if that's what you're looking for.

Artificial Sweeteners Ain't Much Better

How about "Diet cola?" By now you probably know what's coming next. In my opinion, diet soda also needs to be stricken from your nutrition plan. You see, the artificial sweeteners found in diet soda, diet energy drinks, sugar-free sports drinks and other diet drinks may be no better for you than white sugar or high-fructose corn syrup.[23] In fact, some studies suggest that they may be even worse.[24] Artificial sweeteners include aspartame and neotame (Nutra Sweet), sucralose (Splenda), and saccharin (Sweet and Low) and even Stevia (ironically derived from a plant and often marketed as a healthy sugar substitute). Too many product safety tests of these sugar substitutes, although contested by their manufacturers, find possible links to adverse health issues.[25] At best, research and long-term testing of these commonly used artificially synthesized compounds is inconclusive.

The US Food and Drug Administration has approved all of the above artificial sweeteners for human consumption. But are you really going to trust the FDA with your long-term health and well being? I'm not. Is there such a thing as a non-politically influenced government agency? I don't believe so. The same elected representatives who are unable to balance our national budget or put a dent in our looming national debt problem are also responsible for overseeing the FDA.

Am I going to trust another toothless government agency with my health? Not a snowball's chance in hell.

Here's the problem with those artificial sweeteners: they are so good at what they do that they trick your body into behaving as if you're consuming real sugar.[26] They are by definition mimicking the sweet taste of real sugar. Effectively, artificial sweeteners are fooling your taste buds. Makes sense right? This chemistry trick allows food and drink manufacturers to create and sell sweet tasting products with very low or even zero calories. But it's not only your taste buds that are getting fooled. Artificial sweeteners may also be fooling other important functions like your insulin release system. Once again you're messing with the very sensitive hormone insulin and its release system. This affects your normal glycogen storage as well as your appetite. Studies have also shown that people who drink artificially sweetened sodas with meals end up consuming more calories in those meals,[27] and of course you know now what happens to those calories consumed when the body has an insulin spike? Yup. Fat storage. So now you know why I'm preaching the gospel against artificially sweetened foods and drinks.

What You *Should* Drink to Lose Fat

I'm going to let you in on one of the best-kept fitness secrets of all. There is one thing you can drink that will make you feel better, make your body function better and help you lose fat. What is this magic drink? Water. Yes, good old boring water. Water is king. Water is not only a critical component in most bodily functions it keeps you hydrated and helps you flush your system of toxins.[28] Additionally, drinking plenty of water also helps keep your metabolism running a little faster which will help you lose weight faster.[29] It's also calorie free, which means you aren't consuming empty calories.

Tea is also great a great beverage choice. Tea is not only cleansing, it's great source of caffeine. Only drink unsweetened tea made from the plant *Camellia sinensis* which includes black tea, green tea, oolong tea and white tea. Other plant infusions marketed as "herbal teas" are not teas.

So drink water, tea, and coffee. By coffee I mean black coffee not a venti Crappucino containing more sugar than a can of soda or a candy bar. Especially drink lots of water. I'm a huge fan. A sad testament to our society's sugar dependency can be demonstrated with a little experiment. Go to any grocery store and try to find a bottle of unsweetened tea. Heck, walk down the beverage aisle at all your favorite grocery stores and try to find *any* drink at all that contains no sugar *and* no artificial sweetener. I dare you. What you will find is enough sugar-loaded drinks to fatten a large herd of cattle. You'll also find enough artificially sweetened drinks to poison all the lab rats and rhesus monkeys in every R&D lab in corporate America. What you'll be hard pressed to find is a single unsweetened drink, even tea. If I'm lucky I sometimes find one or two unsweetened drinks, about twelve square inches of shelf space at the most. It's a sad state of affairs we're in indeed. The bottom line is, don't drink sugary beverages or artificially sweetened ones. Drink lots of water, unsweetened tea, or black coffee.

Choose Low Glycemic Over High Glycemic Foods

The glycemic index is a measure of our body's rise and change in blood glucose level after eating a food. Foods are ranked based on the rate and the magnitude of their effect on blood glucose or blood sugar. Foods like russet potatoes, sweet potatoes, corn, watermelon, bananas and grapes that are high in sugar are at the high end of the glycemic index scale. The sugar found in vegetables and fruits is bound in fiber so it does not cause an insulin spike, nevertheless, these foods do contain a lot of sugar. As previously explained, if it's not burned immediately this blood sugar will be stored as fat. You can in fact get fat eating potatoes, bananas, oranges and apples. Until you've reached your weight loss goal, I strongly recommend that you eat very limited root vegetables like potatoes and that you don't eat fruit. Once you've reached your fat loss target and you are only working on building lean muscle, then you can add fruit back into your nutrition plan, for example as your pre-workout energy source. I recommend eating fruit just before a cardio session, a strength-training workout or first thing in the morning when you are starting your day and likely to be very active. This helps to ensure the sugar is burned off and not stored as fat.

At the low end of the glycemic index scale are foods whose sugar content is slow to break down. These foods include nuts, green vegetables and whole grains. Low glycemic foods are great for a slow release of energy throughout the day. In terms of carbohydrate rich foods, the distinction between high glycemic and low glycemic foods is essentially another way of saying simple carbohydrates and complex carbohydrates. Put another way, one is immediately available energy and the other is a slow release of energy.

There is no perfect definition of a simple carbohydrate and a complex carbohydrate, because many foods fall somewhere in between. We hear these terms frequently because people like to throw around these labels. For simplicity I will refer to all processed carbohydrates like table sugar and white flour as simple carbohydrates. Complex carbs are whole food sources of carbohydrates, including green vegetables, root vegetables like potatoes, whole grains and legumes. Complex carbohydrates should be your preferred source of energy. Most of the time you'll be relying on low glycemic index food sources for energy. Moderate portions of low glycemic foods are what our bodies are perfectly designed to digest for a slow sustained release of energy.

An easy way to think of the difference between simple and complex carbohydrates is that simple carbs provide a fast burn whereas complex carbs provide a slow burn. Consuming the fast burn type results in an insulin spike, short-lived sugar high and subsequent energy crash (not to mention fat storage). Eating the slow-burn type results in a moderate insulin release triggering a normal absorption of glucose into your muscle cells, fat cells and liver. This provides a slow sustained release of energy over the course of several hours. Our bodies are best equipped to deal with complex carbohydrates for this kind of healthy, sustained energy.

Sugar Is Sugar

As we talk about sugar, one thing I want to reiterate is that as you work towards your fat loss goal, I recommend limiting your fruit consumption. Why? Because intact whole fruit, although rich in fiber and micronutrients including Vitamin A, C, E, beta-carotene, minerals and other beneficial antioxidants, contains a lot of sugar. You'll see in Chapter 7, where we construct meals plans, that for optimal results, most of your calories will come from proteins and fats rather than from carbohydrates. Whether the sugar you eat comes from an apple, orange, banana, raw organic cane sugar, refined white table sugar, a candy bar, a cola drink or even high fructose corn syrup - it's still sugar. To be sure, avoiding the insulin spikes by avoiding sugar is critical for fat loss. And in terms of total calories consumed and compiling the macronutrient ratios within your meal plans, sugar in any form represents a lot of calories from carbohydrates.

An important distinction needs to be made between sugar that naturally occurs in fruits and vegetables, and added sugar, most often refined white sugar. Naturally occurring sugar found in fruits and root vegetables, such as apples and potatoes, is bound in fiber and won't cause the insulin spikes that we're at all times trying to avoid. Added sugar, either in the form of white (table) sugar (sucrose) or high fructose corn syrup is the culprit in wreaking havoc on our insulin release system. Common white sugar, most often made from sugar cane or beets, is made up of 50% glucose and 50% fructose. High fructose corn syrup (HFCS for short) is corn syrup that has undergone a process that converts some of corn's glucose into fructose to produce a desired sweetness. The most common HFCS used in food products such as soft drinks and baked goods is very close to white table sugar in its composition of glucose and fructose. Essentially, chemically, and in its effect on our insulin release system, HFCS is no different than ordinary white table sugar. HFCS is sometimes perceived as somehow worse for us than ordinary table sugar and is often demonized for economic, ethical, and political reasons. First, big agro producers extract it from cheap government subsidized corn reserves. Second, the price of HFCS is held cheap relative to sugar because of US government tariffs on imported sugar, making it a popular sugar substitute. Whatever your own reasons are for avoiding high fructose corn syrup; political, ethical or other, my point is that its effect on our insulin release system is no different then common white table sugar. HFCS is also very cheap to make, thus its popularity as a sweetener in food products. Just remember from a pure fat storage perspective, added sugar and HFCS elicit the same reaction by our body's insulin release system.

So, eating whole fruit containing sugar bound in fiber is much better for you than eating any food with added sugar whether the added sugar is white sugar or high fructose corn syrup. But this doesn't mean you have a free pass to eat all the fruit you want. I've seen people make the mistake of replacing the sweetened junk food or candy bars they used to eat with lots of fruit. Even though they were eating a healthier form of sugar, sugar bound in fiber, they were still consuming a lot of calories as simple carbohydrates, and they had a hard time losing fat.

I'm not saying fruit is unhealthy nor should you stop eating fruit for life. However, if you're serious about losing weight, your nutrition plan should include as close to zero sugar as possible. Temporarily ignore the health benefits of fruit until you've achieved your weight loss goal. As an alternative to fruit you should be eating a variety of green leafy vegetables as well as taking a high quality vitamin & mineral supplement daily. A high quality vitamin and mineral supplement, either in pill form or in a high absorption liquid form is great health insurance.

Now, when you do eat fruit, pick something from the low end of the glycemic index. Cherries, blueberries, raspberries, strawberries, and other berries are best. But again, beware of clever marketing. The overpriced Tibetan goji berries found in your local "health food" store or organic farmers markets are probably no better for you than ordinary garden blueberries. Grown in the Himalayan Mountains sounds exotic and even somehow mystical but they are no richer in antioxidants than blueberries grown in your own backyard. Berries, cherries and grapefruit are also good low glycemic fruit choices.

Here's another marketing warning for you to be aware of. Hand-picked organic one hundred percent pure blue agave nectar is no easier on your waistline than ordinary processed white sugar. "Organic cane sugar" may be good marketing copy when printed on a food product label, but your body's insulin response is no different whether it's organic cane sugar or white table sugar. Some of the big soft drink manufacturing companies have even re-marketed their colas by switching back to using cane sugar instead of HFCS as a sweetener. They're marketing this return to sweetening their popular soft drink brands with sugar as opposed to

HFCS implying that it's now somehow better and healthier. It's not. Added sugar is added sugar. I strongly recommend that you get in the habit of reading labels and don't eat or drink anything that contains added sugar.

Juices and Smoothies

I've also got to add a quick word about juicing and smoothies. Fresh fruit and vegetable juice has become very popular in recent years. Juice bars are becoming a common feature in natural and organic grocery store chains. In many cities fresh juice bars are thriving as stand-alone businesses. In addition, a lot of folks juice and/or blend their own fresh fruit and vegetable shakes at home. Stuff a bunch of fresh kale, spinach, apples, oranges, carrots, and other fruit and vegetables in a blender or juicer and you've got a convenient super healthy drink. Right? Well, kind of but not so fast. Drinking fresh fruit and vegetable smoothies is a great way to get a lot of vitamins, minerals, antioxidants and other micronutrients to be sure. The problem is the sharp blades from a blender destroy the fiber and in the case of juicing the fiber is thrown away. In either case you're consuming sugar devoid of fiber. Sugar, even from fresh fruit, that is no longer bound in fiber will cause that insulin spike we've been talking about. From the perspective of your insulin release system's response, you might as well be drinking a can of cola. Therefore, avoid drinking fruit juices, whether it's fresh squeezed, in a bottle or as part of a smoothie.

What may even be more destructive than the fat storage and the short-term sugar buzz and subsequent energy crash cycles caused by eating added sugar are the long-term health consequences. Continually flooding your body with over-doses of insulin may very well be putting you on the path towards metabolic syndrome like type II diabetes, obesity, high blood pressure, heart disease, dementia, and other associated health problems. By now you know a big part of the solution. Read labels carefully and don't eat anything with added sugar.

Talk about beating a dead horse, I've exhausted the topic of sugar. I do sincerely hope that I've made one thing clear. Refined carbohydrates like white flour and sugar are processed poisons. Don't pick up another syringe. Get off the smack, no more heroin. Refined carbohydrates have zero nutritional value and can lead to serious health issues. Stop ingesting these poisons. Don't eat white sugar, white flour or any other refined carbohydrates.

If you were given a new Ferrari, would you run your million dollar sports car on used cooking oil you found in a dumpster behind a fast food restaurant? Hell no, you'd fill it up on the highest quality racing fuel only. Treat your body with the same respect and care. Your body is much more valuable than any sports car. It's also the only body you'll ever have.

Enough about what we should not be eating. Let's move on now and talk about the foods we should be eating.

Chapter 4

"Fit feels better than any food tastes."

- Unknown

The Right Fuel to Get Fit and Lean

Food is fuel. It and can either be medicinal or toxic. Food is medicine or food is poison. Nothing is neutral. Putting it in those terms makes it pretty easy to choose what you eat wisely, I think. We've established that joining the herd and following the lemmings over the cliff is a bad idea. Eating the readily available mass-produced processed garbage that surrounds us will plump you up, cause countless health problems and eventually kill you. So **what is** the right fuel? I'm only putting the cleanest fuel I can get my hands on in my body. I strongly suggest you do the same.

Here's the not so terribly complicated secret: Eat nutrient-rich fresh <u>intact whole foods</u>. That's it. ***Eat lean proteins, healthy fats, and intact whole food*** *sources of carbohydrates coming mostly from green vegetables along with limited amounts of root vegetables, whole grains, and fruits.*

A couple of grocery shopping tips for you to live by courtesy of Michael Pollan, author of *The Omnivore's Dilemma*.

1. <u>Try to buy items only from the outer perimeter of the grocery store.</u>

Fresh foods, most of which need refrigeration, tend to be located around the perimeter of the store. The interior of the store is generally filled with food-like products that are loaded with salt, preservatives and artificial ingredients to ensure extended shelf life. They're also easy to recognize because they're packaged in a box or a can. These items should not be eaten by anyone following the Get Fit, Lean program.

2. <u>Always read the nutrition label.</u>

Labels give you lots of information you need including calories and the ratio and amounts of protein/carbs/fats. Labels even tell you how much fiber vs sugar is in each serving. This is important, especially whether or not there is added sugar. Avoid everything with added sugar. The other thing labels must list is all of the artificial additives and chemical compounds that have been added to the "food." Pollan's rule for that is: don't buy anything that your grandmother wouldn't recognize as food. Long lists of unpronounceable chemical compounds are a dead giveaway for processed foods, refined foods, manufactured fats, and other chemical additives. Simple rules I think. Put these two simple rules into practice and it's hard to go too terribly wrong.

Meat: It's What's for Breakfast, Lunch, and Dinner

Like a lion, tiger or wolf, I like to consider myself a large carnivore. Ok, in reality I'm an omnivore, but that just doesn't sound as cool. What I mean is, I'm a meat eater. I love most everything off the hoof. Growing up in the Midwest I learned to love eating about any meat grilled over an open flame. Grilled fresh vegetables, prepared well, can be delicious and satisfying as well. Regarding the question of whether or not we humans were ever intended to live as vegetarians, I defer to the wisdom of the well-known television celebrity, life coach and philosopher, Homer J. Simpson. Homer so eloquently once said, "If God had wanted us to be vegetarians he wouldn't have made all of the animals out of meat."

If you choose to be a vegetarian then you're likely getting the majority of your protein from soy bean-based sources like tofu, bean curd or soy milk and products. Eating tofu has been shown to increase the effects of estrogen[30], the female sex hormone, in your body.[31] The male sex hormone testosterone promotes increased muscle and bone mass, not estrogen. If eating soy is your strategy for building lean muscle, I wish you the best of luck. No single vegetable is a complete protein. This means no vegetable contains all the essential amino acids. Eat only vegetables and you may not be getting all the essential amino acids, the building blocks of protein.

Understandably, there are those who choose not to eat animal products for humane or other personal reasons. I respect that philosophy although my Get Fit, Lean program focuses on animal proteins. I recognize that if you combine enough vegetables it is possible to get all the essential amino acids. However, doing so requires quite a number of different veggies to build a complete protein meal. Trying to build lean muscle as a vegetarian is challenging, and I wish the vegetarians all the best. If you are not a vegetarian, then I recommend eating eggs, fish, and meat. Even if you do choose to source your protein from plants instead of animals, I think you will still find the rest of my book useful to get fit and lean.

The Three Macronutrients

Let's begin building your nutrition plan by grouping all foods into the three basic macronutrient groups. These are (1) proteins, (2) fats and (3) carbohydrates. At the simplest level your nutrition will be made up of just three rules.

Rule #1 is eat the correct amount of total calories.

Rule #2 is eat the correct proportion or ratio of macros from each of the three groups.

Rule #3 is to eat the right foods from each of the three macronutrient groups.

I'll tell you about a handy online tool and app to help you keep track of calories, macronutrients, and foods soon in another chapter. Right now, let's talk about what foods you *should* be eating from these three macronutrient groups.

Macronutrient 1: Lean Proteins

As noted previously, protein is essential for building and maintaining muscle and will be a key staple of your nutrition plan. The majority of your calories will come from protein. The best sources of lean protein are egg whites, poultry white meat, fish, and lean red meat.

Egg whites are nature's purest whole food source of low-fat high-protein nutrition. The possible negative effects of the high cholesterol content of egg yolk is debatable. Regardless of whether or not too much cholesterol may be bad for you, egg yolk is very high in fat and fat is the most calorie dense macronutrient. This fat represents a lot of calories, so from the perspective of weight loss through a calorie-controlled nutrition plan, you're better off *not* eating the egg yolk. You have a certain number of calories available to consume every day and you can make better use of your available calories. So skip the egg yolks but do make use of nature's perfect protein source, egg whites.

So what *should* you eat? Here's a good example of a meal that provides high-quality lean protein: a breakfast egg-white scramble. I use six egg whites in my egg white scramble every morning. Add two to three ounces of diced chicken breast, half an avocado, and some chili sauce or your favorite hot sauce. Then add a slice of whole grain toast and it becomes a hearty, healthy, high-protein meal complete with the best source of fiber-rich healthy fat as well, avocado. This meal is delicious. It just might be my favorite meal of the day. There's something very satisfying to me about avocados and hot sauce. The rich fat content tastes so decadent it's almost as if I'm cheating on my nutrition plan. But it's not cheating - it's a very healthy meal. This meal is high in lean protein, rich in healthy fat, fiber, and complex (low glycemic) carbohydrates. It's a perfect breakfast made up entirely of clean sources of each of the three macronutrients.

White meat poultry is also a great source of protein. Chicken and turkey is the most common, but try to avoid the dark meat and stick with the breast. Turkey white meat is generally leaner than chicken white meat, but both are very lean compared to most other meat sources. The difference between chicken and turkey is not really significant, so it doesn't matter which one you choose – both are excellent choices. One great thing about yard bird is the many different ways that you can cook it. You can BBQ (using a healthy spice rub, not a sweet sugary BBQ sauce), grill, bake, broil or stir fry it, just don't deep-fry your chicken. If you stir-fry your chicken, choose a clean cooking oil with no hydrogenated oil. Good choices are olive, sunflower or saffron oil. Cooking hint: chicken breast needs a little flavor help. A tasty marinade sauce or salt (used sparingly) and pepper really helps chicken. Lawry's Seasoning Salt could become your new best friend in the kitchen. Just be careful about using rubs and marinades, because many rubs, marinades and seasonings contain added sugar and a lot of salt. So once again, I recommend that you read the nutrition labels and buy only those with no added sugar. Also, go easy on the salt – a little bit goes a long way.

Speaking of that, I'd like to mention a quick word about sodium or as it's more commonly known, salt. If most of your calories come from fresh intact whole foods as opposed to processed food-like products packaged in a box or a can, you're probably not overdoing the salt. However, as I just mentioned, many seasonings, marinades, and rubs are loaded with salt. Excess salt can lead to high blood pressure as well as other adverse health issues including heart and kidney problems. The average adult only needs about 1,500 mg of salt per day, but most Americans consume more than twice that amount. Once again, reading labels is important.

Ok, back to protein sources. Fish are also a great source of lean protein. One great thing about fish is the wide variety of choices to pick from. White fish have less oils than do cold water fish like salmon, mackerel, sardines and anchovies. Although higher in calories, oil-rich fish like salmon is a great source of omega-3 fatty acids. Omega-3s are a type of fat that you should be eating regularly. White fish generally contain the same fatty acid nutrients but in much less quantity than oily fish. Most fish is already rich in flavor, and therefore it needs very little help in terms of seasoning. Add just a dash of salt and pepper, a squeeze of lemon juice, a dash of olive oil or a splash of white wine. Baked, grilled or pan fried (pan fried recipes should use just a tablespoon of healthy cooking oil in a skillet), fish is delicious and a great source of high quality protein.

Another fish option that in my humble opinion is the tastiest of all is sashimi. I'm not talking about sushi rolls loaded with white rice, mayo, friend tempura and who knows what else. I'm talking about nothing but high quality fresh fish. It isn't exactly the most economical protein option, but if you can afford it once in a while, sashimi is a great protein source.

Red meat is another great source of animal protein although it is often and unfairly demonized for its animal fat (saturated fat) content. So there are a couple things to consider when eating red meat to ensure you're not overdoing it on the fats. By weight, fats are more calorie dense than proteins and carbs; therefore, in order not to exceed your total daily calories from fat target, you will want to eat the leanest cut you can afford. Not all cuts of the cow are created equally. Tenderloin filets are your best choice when minimizing the fat, but other cuts like a skirt steak and flank steak aren't bad either. Because red meat is so calorie-dense due to the fat content, eat it in moderation and in reasonable portions. Don't become famous for getting your name carved on the wall at Big Billy Bob's Sizzlin' Steak Barn by putting away the 64-oz NY strip. A five- to seven-ounce filet is all you need for a single meal's serving of protein.

Many traditional "health and nutrition experts" as well as those in the medical community still advise us to limit our red meat consumption. So, should you avoid red meat or let your carnivore instincts run wild? Numerous studies have shown that the highest correlation to heart disease is not red meat consumption (nor animal fats, *ie,* saturated fats in general) but rather heredity[32]. If you've got a family history of heart disease, you too are most likely predisposed to the same trouble. If there is no history of heart disease in your family, then you most likely have much less risk. That said, I'm not a cardiologist. The prudent thing to do is to go see a doctor and get a physical exam with a complete blood work. Speak to your doctor and learn your family history. Some people get away with consuming as much animal fat as they like and some don't. If you are not predisposed to heart disease, then a few servings of red meat per week or even once a day is a good way to diversify your protein consumption. Red meat also provides large amounts of

B-12, iron, and zinc. If red meat is not for you, no worries, there are plenty of other protein sources.

As a healthy happy omnivore, I believe animal proteins should be your primary source of protein. From the perspective of a calorie controlled nutrition plan, eggs whites, chicken breast and fish are the best sources. Only animal proteins contain all the essential amino acids in the right proportions. No single plant based protein does. Essential amino acids cannot be synthesized within the human body so must be consumed via the food we eat. Amino acids are the building blocks of proteins, which in turn are the building blocks of muscle tissue. My recommendation is to eat meat.

What about soy? Unlike other plant or vegetable proteins, soy protein does contain all the essential amino acids.[33] Soy proteins such as bean curd and tofu are relatively low-fat high protein alternatives to protein from meat however two of the nine essential amino acids only occur in small amounts. As mentioned earlier, you can build complete proteins by combining the right vegetables. However in the case of soy, given the possible increased effects of estrogen, I steer clear of it just in case.

Macronutrient 2: Healthy Fats

First of all, you may be asking, what's the difference between unhealthy and healthy fats? For decades, government public health organizations and established medicine doctrine has taught us that consuming saturated fats leads to heart disease and other health problems. The conventional wisdom, as well as American Heart Association (AHA) dogma, is that saturated fats are unhealthy and unsaturated fats are healthy.[34] Ever since the now very questionable validity of the 1955 study, "Seven Countries Study" by Ancel Keys, who went on to sit on and influence the AHA nutrition committee, the American public has been led to believe bad science. The AHA dogma teaches that eating too much animal fats including butter, lard, egg (yolk), and red meat leads to coronary disease.[35] Several recent studies have turned this idea on its head. Much of the latest research tells us that consuming animal fat *does not* correlate to coronary disease.[36] As a consequence of US Government health and nutrition agencies perpetuating bad science, and the food industry's campaign to remove saturated fats from our diet beginning in the early 1960s, we've swapped (saturated) fats for refined carbohydrates. Hence the still popular "low fat" or "fat free" marketing labels found on so many food-like products. Saturated fats (mostly animal fats), which as it turns out may not be bad for us at all, have been removed and replaced with simple carbohydrates that most certainly cause multiple health problems.[37] Eating fat doesn't necessarily make you fat, but eating sugar and flour will not only expand your waistline, eating refined carbohydrates will also put you on the road to metabolic syndrome.

The AHA frames their argument against eating saturated fats like this. Saturated fatty acids stimulate your liver to produce more low-density lipoproteins (LDLs, also frequently called "bad cholesterol") whereas unsaturated fatty acids cause your liver to produce more high-density lipoproteins (HDLs, also called "good cholesterol"). Consuming foods high in LDLs has long been associated with heart disease. Conversely, consuming foods high in HDLs has long been associated with reducing risk factors associated with cardiovascular disease.[38] However, more recent studies have shown that it's much more complicated than the AHA suggests. There are two variations of LDLs, type A and type B. Type A, the small dense LDL, is the "bad" cholesterol. The most prevalent one, type B, the large buoyant LDL is thought to be "neutral" from a cardiovascular standpoint. Type A, the bad LDL is increased by consumption of carbohydrates.[39]

I believe the healthy fats versus unhealthy fats discussion should be framed as natural fats, both saturated and unsaturated, versus manufactured fats. The true bad fat that should definitely be avoided is trans fat. Hydrogenated oil, although technically an oil and not a fat, should also be avoided. Both are proven to cause health multiple problems.[40] Trans fat consumption has been implicated in heart disease, stroke, diabetes, and other chronic conditions.[41] Trans fat does occur naturally in very small quantities, however most of it used in food products is created artificially. Trans fat is a solid at 98.6 degrees Fahrenheit, our internal temperature. How creepy is that? Our bodies cannot metabolize trans fat because it's more closely related to plastic than food. You should have a zero tolerance for trans fat.

So, is it all right eat both unsaturated *and* saturated fats? Yes, as long as they are naturally occurring as opposed to manufactured. However, you do need to consider your total available calories for consumption. All fat, both saturated and unsaturated, is calorie dense: 1 gram of fat has 9 calories, whereas 1 gram of protein as well as 1 gram of carbohydrate has 4 calories each. This means that in terms managing a calorie controlled nutrition plan, you're not going to be eating a whole lot of fats anyway. I love red meat. I particularly enjoy a good steak for dinner or other red meats in reasonable portions but don't eat it more than once a day because of the calorie impact on my nutrition plan.

A clear distinction can be drawn between saturated and unsaturated fat. Although high in iron and other minerals, red meat is void of fiber. By comparison, the humble little avocado is an excellent source of dietary fiber as well as vitamins and minerals. Another great source of unsaturated fat also high in dietary fiber is almonds. If you compare equal weights of cooked chicken breast to cooked read meat you'll find that chicken has more protein, less calories, and less fat. If the majority of your protein comes from lean sources such as chicken breast, eggs whites and white fish, then you'll have more calories to eat unsaturated fat sources like avocado and almonds that contain valuable dietary fiber.

Nuts like almonds and walnuts to name a few, cold water oily fish, and avocados are, in my opinion, the best whole food sources of fats. I eat half an avocado and 1 to 2 oz of nuts everyday. It doesn't matter if you eat raw or roasted nuts, the nutritional value is the same. Although the salted varieties usually do taste better, they should be avoided because of their sodium content. Why? Water retention.

It's worth including a note about salt. Salt is one mineral that most people usually consume many multiples the amount we actually need. Salt does have value. It improves the taste of most foods and it's an excellent preservative. This is why you'll find that so many of the food-like products packaged in cans or boxes are loaded with salt. The problem is that consuming too much salt will make you retain water. Our bodies are very efficient machines, always trying to achieve equilibrium. If you saturate yourself with more salt than you need, you'll hold water, feel bloated and carry around extra-unwanted pounds. In addition, that extra water causes your heart to work harder and contributes to conditions like high blood pressure. That's why it's important for people with high blood pressure to reduce their salt intake. Skipping the table salt is a good start, although the reality is that most sodium in the average person's diet comes from packaged, processed foods.[42] If you follow my Get Fit, Lean nutrition plan, most of your meals will come from fresh intact whole food sources so too much salt will no longer be an issue.

Let's get back to talking about avocados. As I previously mentioned, a delicious way to add avocado to your meal plan is to scoop out half of the little green fruit and then rest it gently on top of your favorite breakfast egg scramble with a splash of hot sauce. Another great tasting avocado dish is slicing them up on a bed of spinach salad with just a bit of balsamic vinegar and olive oil. The avocado absorbs the balsamic and olive oil, which tastes delicious. Raw avocado slices on top of baked chicken breast taste great as well. Another delicious suggestion is adding avocado slices to a roast chicken or turkey sandwich made with whole grain bread.

Cold water oily fish like salmon, herring, mackerel, anchovies and sardines are not only great protein sources but very high in the essential fatty acid, omega 3. Eating at least a couple of servings of oily fish per week is a very healthy habit to get into, so I strongly recommended including oily fish in your meal plan. These types of fish are easy to prepare and have great flavor on their own. They need very little seasoning help if any at all to taste great. Baked salmon with just a dash of lemon juice and a pinch of ground pepper is my favorite.

Macronutrient 3: Carbohydrates

Much digital ink has been spilled in my discussion of the ill effects of processed carbohydrates. But this is not to say that all carbohydrates are bad. Although we are able to obtain most of our energy requirements from proteins and fats, whole intact carbohydrates are a good source of energy as well. Whole food sources of complex carbohydrates low on the glycemic index are best. Dietary fiber (sometimes known as roughage) is an indigestible form of carbohydrate, and is also beneficial in maintaining good health.

The meal plan that is going to help you shed weight most effectively is a low carbohydrate plan. You will not be eating simple carbohydrates from sugar nor any refined flour. Instead, the majority of your carbs will come from fresh green vegetables and limited amounts of root vegetables and whole grains.

Carbs from Fresh Fruits

Fresh fruits are great for you. Fresh fruits are nutrient rich natural whole foods. Fruits are high in micronutrients like vitamin C and other important vitamins and minerals, antioxidants and fiber. Unfortunately, as I discussed earlier, most fruits also very high in our nemesis. Wait for it, sugar! From the perspective of a calorie controlled nutrition plan, sugar is high in calories. Whether the source is an apple, banana, orange, organic raw cane sugar or ordinary white table sugar, it's adding a lot of calories to your meal plan. Those calories can me better utilized for proteins and fats. If your goal is to lose weight, I recommend that you don't eat fruit, and get your vitamins and minerals elsewhere. You can add fruit back into your nutrition plan after you've reached your goal weight and are in maintenance mode.

If you're a skinny person looking to simply add muscle, fresh fruits are a good energy source when eaten in moderation. You must consider fruit a small portion of your daily carbohydrate consumption. Don't have more than a couple of pieces a day. I recommend eating fresh fruit just before, during or just after a workout. Fresh fruit is good source of workout energy fuel as it's both easily and quickly digested. Fruit is a natural source of sugar so use it as natural workout fuel for energy.

There are a wide variety of fruits available, so mix it up. Try different kinds. Eat an apple or an orange on one day then on another day try a grapefruit or a banana. Eat different varieties of fruits as they all have a slightly different composition of vitamins and minerals. For the best flavor, stick with the local seasonal choices as much as possible. Ripening fruit on the vine in the sun, as opposed to in a container on a cargo ship steaming half way around the world or a semi truck carrying it across the country, usually makes a huge difference in taste. Sun ripened equates to delicious; ship ripened, not so much.

Carbs from Fresh Vegetables

Mom always said, "Eat your vegetables." Mom was right. For the sake of this discussion we'll divide all vegetables into just two groups. The two groups are (1) leafy green or other colorful veggies grown above ground and (2) root vegetables. If you ever absolutely have to pig out on some kind of food, then make green vegetables your vice. Veggies like broccoli, asparagus, cauliflower, green beans, pea pods, spinach, kale, summer squash, zucchini and the seemingly endless varieties of dark greens are typically rich in vitamins and minerals and fiber but very low in calories. Apart from root vegetables like potatoes and carrots, they also contain pretty much zero sugar across the board. Pile the green veggies on your plate; they're good for you, low in calories, and can help satisfy your appetite when you're hungry.

Some of the popular old school "healthy cookbooks" and "diet books" will recommend that you steam your vegetables. This is certainly an option, but in my opinion, it usually makes them taste really bland. Steaming too long will also purge most of the nutrients out of your fresh veggies and into the boiling water only to get poured down the drain.[43] If you do steam your veggies make it real quick and at a high temperature. A quick steam locks in the nutrients as well as keeps them crisp and tasty. I prefer to grill or bake my veggies. One easy method for grilling or baking is to first cut them up then toss them in a large plastic freezer/storage bag. Add a dash of salt and pepper or seasoning salt, some crushed red pepper (if you like spicy foods) and a tablespoon of olive oil and then shake up the bag. Empty the bag onto a BBQ grill or a cookie sheet and grill or bake for fifteen to twenty minutes at 375 degrees. I think this method is especially tasty with asparagus, broccoli, squash and brussel sprouts.

Other than in the case of potatoes, eating your veggies raw is also a good option. This ensures getting the micronutrients in their intact whole natural form. Some argue that the chemical structure of the vegetables' nutrients is altered through the heating process, thereby degrading their value significantly. This is true to a degree in the case of certain vegetables, so do try to include raw vegetables in your meal plan. Tossed salads are a great way to consume raw vegetables as well as get some beneficial fiber. Add tomato, cucumber, onions, bell peppers and so on to your favorite types of lettuce. Just don't use the lettuce as a placeholder for a decadent creamy salad dressing that can turn a low fat healthy meal into a giant calorie bomb. I love the classic blue cheese wedge found on the menu at most good steak house across the USA as much as the next guy, but it's really just a giant calorie delivery mechanism. Give up the blue cheese wedge. Your best bet for salad dressing is mixing olive oil and balsamic vinegar. This is best because you get your greens, some veggies, fiber and healthy omega-6 fat from the olive oil. If you've got to have dressing out of a bottle find a low fat low sugar variety. Read the label. If there are more than a couple of grams of sugar per serving then it's not a good choice for helping you get fit and lean.

Root vegetables are a great whole food source of complex carbohydrates. Baked sweet potatoes might just be every bodybuilding, physique, figure and bikini competitor's go-to carbohydrate of choice. Sweet potatoes are nature's perfect whole food source of sustained clean energy. Additionally, sweet potatoes are also easy to prepare. They can be thrown straight in the oven and baked or microwaved and still taste great hot or cold with nothing added. Acquire a taste for sweet potatoes. This perfect complex carbohydrate source will serve you well.

A common misunderstanding is the difference between sweet potatoes and yams. Grocery stores often mislabel different varieties of sweet potato varieties as yams when they are not really yams at all. True yams are not root vegetables, and instead grow on vines – but they are still very low in sugar and a good choice for your complex carb needs. Admittedly, this may be a botanical distinction that is only interesting to me.

White, gold, red, and yellow potatoes are also a good whole food source of complex carbohydrate but slightly higher on the glycemic index scale (see below) than sweet potatoes. Compared head to head sweet potatoes come out as a better choice. Sweet potatoes are higher in Vitamin A, have more vitamin C, more fiber and fewer total carbs than white potatoes.

Carbs from Whole Grains

Whole grains are an excellent source of the right kind of complex, slow-burning carbohydrates. However, many people confuse **whole grains** with other types of multi-grains or whole wheat products. Whole grain bread is something very different from wheat bread, brown bread and even from whole wheat bread. Read the nutrition label. If it doesn't say **whole grain** then it's made from some refined grain. Marketers are very clever and often misleading, trying to make foods sound healthier than they are. The nutritional ingredients label must say **whole grain**. A true whole grain's cereal germ, endosperm and bran are intact. Whole grains are a great source of complex carbohydrates as opposed to refined grains, which are processed flours akin to white sugar. Brown bread and often wheat bread are just marketing verbiage intended to make bread appear healthy when in fact it's no healthier than ordinary white bread. Don't eat food products made from refined grains. They differ from the ordinary white bread we ate on our PB&Js as kids only in name and color. Eating breads made from anything other than whole grains will cause the unwanted insulin spike. Your body's response to eating bread made from refined flour is not very different from eating a bag of candy or any other processed sugar.

Whole grains, on the other hand, are complex carbohydrates. They provide energy to fuel you for sustained periods of time. There are a variety of whole grains to choose from including wheat, oats, barley, brown rice, farro, rye, millet, quinoa, and buckwheat to name just a few. Some food products made from whole grains include whole-grain flour, whole-grain bread, whole-grain pasta and rolled oats/ oatmeal. Just be careful when reading the labels to be sure it notes that it was made from whole grains. One thing to remember about oatmeal is to buy and eat the kind with no added sugar or other flavorings. Sweetened brown maple sugar oatmeal may not be much better for you than chocolate-frosted sugar bombs. Watch out for and avoid whole grain products with added sugar.

My favorite source of whole grain might be oatmeal and oat bran. Whole oats make a great tasting breakfast in the morning and provide an all-day energy source. Add your favorite chocolate protein powder and a couple of tablespoons of natural peanut butter and you've got a complete meal. This delicious combination contains foods from all three macronutrient groups. Oatmeal, protein powder and peanut butter are a great way to start your day. Once you've reached your weight loss target and graduated to the maintenance phase you can then add some blueberries or strawberries on top. Oatmeal is an extremely healthy carbohydrate source providing sustained energy that will fuel your body for hours.

Whole-grain breads are also delicious, especially as there are so many health conscious manufacturers these days. They're good at making breads interesting by combining different whole grains. In addition, whole-grain pastas are a great carbohydrate choice. They are a much better choice than their characterless cousin, fiber-less pasta made from refined flour. Whole-grain pastas may seem a little dense or heavy at first, but after you get accustomed to them, pasta made from refined flour will taste like mush by comparison.

Dairy Products

I'm often asked by people if they should eat any dairy products – and here's my answer. Milk is Mother Nature's perfectly designed food for mammal babies. After we're weaned from our mother's breast milk there is no need to ever have milk again. However, dairy industry lobbyists would love for you to believe otherwise. The truth is milk contains no essential nutrients that can't easily be sourced elsewhere. The dairy industry spends a lot of money advertising milk doing a body good. Often, milk sold at the grocery store is loaded with added sugar or it wouldn't taste so good. Milk also contains lactose (a naturally occurring sugar found in milk) and animal fat. The simple fact is that we should not drink milk as part of the Get Fit, Lean nutrition plan.

There are other problems with adding dairy in your nutrition plan as it relates to fat loss. Cheese and other common dairy products are usually high in saturated (animal) fat, and cheese can be high in sodium. Saturated fat may not be the most efficient type of fat to fuel your body. Additionally, most milk and yogurts sold in grocery stores contain added sugar. As you know by now, the added sugar in milk and other dairy products such as yogurt is going to result in the aforementioned insulin response.

Exceptions to the No Dairy Rule

There are a few notable exceptions to the no dairy rule. Low-fat cottage cheese contains very little fat and no added sugar. It's low in carbohydrates and fat while very high in protein. Unsweetened plain Greek yogurt has a similar nutrition profile to low-fat cottage cheese: very low in fat, contains no added sugar, and is high in protein. Again, my mantra is read the nutrition labels. If you're going to eat any dairy then look for products very low in saturated fat and with no added sugar or salt.

Many protein powder supplements are made from whey and casein, which are both derived from milk. These are acceptable to include in the Get Fit, Lean nutrition plan, but if you are lactose intolerant you may have a negative reaction. Other than these exceptions (cottage cheese, plain yogurt, and whey/casein-based protein powders) I advise you not to eat dairy products.

Gluten

If you're one of the less than 1% of the population who has celiac disease, you should not eat gluten. Gluten is found in grains like wheat, barley and rye. Oats are gluten free. Some people confuse wheat allergies with gluten intolerance. Gluten sensitivity and wheat allergy are two different conditions. But the bottom line is, if you're sensitive or allergic to something then avoid consuming it.

Gluten is a protein composite found in wheat and related grain species. The primary proteins found in gluten are glutenin and gliadin. Most historians believe that humans begin eating wheat about 10,000 years ago with the advent of agriculture. Our digestive systems are unable to fully break down gliadin, a strange indigestible protein. For the small fraction of the population with celiac disease, this causes serious intestinal problems. For everyone else, the undigested protein passes harmlessly through your intestinal tract.

Why are so many food products labeled gluten-free? Labeling foods like bread, cookies, and cake made with any kind of flour as "gluten free" has become a popular marketing fad. Like the popular "fat-free" and "organic" labels stamped on so many food products, a "gluten-free" label also helps sell food products to uneducated consumers who hear about gluten intolerance and jump to the conclusion that gluten is bad. So savvy food marketers realized that "gluten-free" labels could help sell otherwise nondescript foods to unsuspecting people who think it equates to a more healthy food product.

This is not unlike the "war against fat." A few years ago the popular marketing label stamped on many food products was "fat-free." It's still widely used as a marketing ploy to make foods sound healthier than they actually are. I find the fat-free label particularly ironic. Slapping on a fat-free label implies that the food product is somehow healthy, and the marketers want you to think that eating fat-free foods is going to help you control your weight. What fat-free too often really means is they've removed the fat and replaced it with added sugar.[44] The irony is that eating fat doesn't necessarily make you fat; in actuality eating sugar is what makes you fat. You want to get really fat? Eat a lot of packaged and processed "fat-free" foods.

In my opinion, like all popular fads, the gluten-free fad will pass in a few years. If not eating gluten makes you feel better then don't eat gluten. You can easily get all the necessary nutrients you require without eating gluten. For people who don't have wheat allergies and the 140 out of 141 people who don't actually have celiac,[45] the undigested gliadin fragments will usually pass harmlessly through the gut.[46]

Hydration

Continuous hydration is important for all of your body's normal functions. Hydration is also critical for peak athletic performance. If you don't drink enough water, you'll end up thirsty, light headed, and lose coordination. Insufficient water consumption will also fatigue your muscles and can cause cramping. Without adequate water your body loses its ability to cool itself, which can lead to heat exhaustion, and in extreme, situations, even death.

As I mentioned previously in the section about what you *should* be drinking, water consumption is a little-known weight loss secret. First, drinking enough water throughout the day can curb your appetite because it makes you feel fuller. When you feel fuller, you eat less. Drinking water also sparks your body to produce more heat. Your body heats the water you drink thereby increasing your metabolism, which in turn helps you burn more calories.[47]

Don't wait until you're thirsty to drink water. Instead, hydrate before you exercise. Your heart doesn't have to work as hard when you are adequately hydrated. Nutrients and oxygen are transported more efficiently to your muscles when you are properly hydrated.

I recommend that you start hydrating one to two hours before you exercise if possible (if you work out first thing in the morning, then begin hydrating when you wake up). An average adult should drink about 16 to 24 ounces of water in the two hour window before exercise then drink about 8 ounces every 15 minutes during your training. If you're doing your cardio outside on a hot day under the sun, you may need much more. You should be replacing the fluids you lose from sweating with water as you exercise. You will improve your performance and help achieve your weight goals by staying hydrated.

What to Eat Summary

You are now armed with good working knowledge of the foods you should be eating and how to choose them. In a later chapter I'll present some menu ideas with accompanying nutrient information. You don't have to wait to start eating clean. Start now. Choose only high quality food items for every meal of the day. The correct portions of foods from the three macronutrient groups will not trigger an insulin spike nor the accompanying energy highs and lows. Start eating the right intact whole foods in reasonable quantities now and you'll experience an immediate benefit. Post-lunch food comas will quickly become a thing of the past. Instead you'll experience sustained energy lasting all day long, and you'll begin losing fat by reducing your processed carbohydrate and sugar intake. Speaking of which, it's time to dig into the right macronutrient portioning to begin building the new you. Ready to supercharge yourself? Let's go!

Chapter 5

"We are what we repeatedly do. Excellence, then, is not an act, but a habit."

- Aristotle

The Right Macronutrient Ratios

In this chapter, I'm going to outline what I consider the optimal macronutrient ratios for you to eat in order to fuel your workouts and turn your body into a fat-burning, muscle-building machine. But first, you may need to unlearn a lot of misinformation that's been "fed" to you since childhood.

In 1943, during World War II, the United States government introduced its first attempt at nutritional guidelines, "The Basic 7." The United States Department of Agriculture (USDA) then recommended the "Basic Four" in 1956. The "Food Guide Pyramid" was introduced in 1992, and most recently "My Plate" in 2011. The US government's latest iteration (My Plate) is starting to approach a reasonably healthy nutrition plan, but once again falls short of good advice. These recommendations are outdated, watered-down notions shaped by politically motivated special interest groups like dairy and meat lobbyists, among others. So forget about the nutrition plans and food pyramids you've been told you should follow. They're largely rubbish. I'm going to share with you a healthy fat loss plan that really works.

Protein, Fat, and Carbohydrates

There are no special interest groups influencing my program. Your single motivation for following my nutrition plan need only be to build a better body. The Get Fit, Lean nutrition plan is intentionally straightforward and easy to follow. Visualize my nutrition plan as a tree diagram or flow chart. It starts with getting your calories under control. You've first got to figure out the right number of calories to consume. If your goal is to lose weight then you'll put yourself in calorie deficit. Second, eat the right mix of macronutrients. This simply means correctly dividing your total calories among the three macronutrient groups of proteins, fats and carbohydrates. Third, eat the right foods within each of the three macronutrient groups. That's it. That is all you have to do.

The Get Fit, Lean Nutrition Plan Basics

Manage Your Calorie Intake
- Determine calorie baseline
- Calorie deficit = weight loss
- Calorie surplus = weight gain

Eat the Right Mix of Macronutrients
- 45% Protein
- 35% Fats
- 20% Carbohydrates

Eat Whole Intact Foods
- Lean protein
- Healthy fats
- Complex carbohydrates

The optimal Get Fit, Lean nutrition plan is that simple. The good news is that all the components of the plan are really easy to track with precision. Free websites and smart phone apps are available to calculate all this for you. They're easy to set up and maintain after entering a few personal details. I'll spell out exactly how to do this in the coming chapter on calorie counting and meal planning.

Changing Your Body Composition

In order to get fit and lean, there are two separate but related problems that you're ultimately going to solve. The first is absolute weight loss or net weight. Let's call it scale weight. You're most likely carrying a few extra pounds so you're going to lose scale weight. Second, you're going to change your body composition, meaning you're going to reduce fat and build lean muscle.

Losing scale weight is pure physics. It's a thermodynamics problem and the solution is found in a very simple formula. It's not complicated, and in fact is very straightforward: consume more calories than you burn and you'll gain weight.

Burn more calories than you consume and you'll lose weight. That's it. Absolute weight loss alone or losing scale weight is a simple enough problem to solve, right? It may seem too simple, and it is.

But the Get Fit, Lean program is not just about losing scale weight. It's about changing your body composition. Now, the solution to the body composition problem is more complicated because it requires doing two seemingly contradictory things simultaneously. You're going to lose and gain at the same time. You will lose fat while you're building muscle. Losing and gaining at the same time is a delicate balance. Success requires the right nutrition plan. As discussed earlier, nutrition is 80% of your transformation. You have to get the total nutrition plan right. If your goal were only weight loss then you'd simply stay in calorie deficit.

We have much loftier goals than merely dropping scale weight: my program is a body transformation guide. We're going to reshape your physique by shedding fat and gaining lean muscle simultaneously. Therefore, scale weight, although a helpful measure of progress, begins to lose much of its importance. Instead, how you look in the mirror and to others, how your clothes fit your newly honed body, and how you feel will tell the real story.

So let's get to it. Exactly how many calories should you eat and what mix of macronutrients you should consume in order to achieve this? Getting this part right is critical. Let's walk through the nutrition plan where I'll address all the relevant questions.

First, you need to know exactly how much you are eating. You need to measure everything you eat. There are two ways to approach tracking what you are eating. I'll begin with a short description of the simple - but not extremely accurate - "eyeball approach." I'll then move on to the highly recommended sophisticated and accurate method, the "dialed in" approach, which I encourage you to stick with.

The Eyeball Approach

Let me share a word about the eyeball estimate, or simple estimation approach. When I did my 12-week body transformation contest in 2009, I lost 30 pounds of scale weight while gaining lean muscle. I was able to achieve this without counting a single calorie. I never weighed a single thing I ate, monitored my heart rate, or kept track of how many calories I burned while doing cardio training. I merely followed some very simple, admittedly crude guidelines and nevertheless achieved great results. In fairness to me, I had never heard of a calorie counting website and at the time and I didn't own a smartphone. If online programs or apps for calorie counting, nutrition planning and workout tracking existed in the spring of 2009, I wasn't aware of them.

Therefore, I don't recommend following the eyeball approach unless you have no other choice. Looking back I now realize I could have done better if I had followed a more sophisticated, measured and planned approach. Since then I've become much more precise and surprisingly found the entire tracking process no more difficult than estimating. There are now simple-to-use, free online tools and smartphone apps available to anyone with an Internet connection or smartphone. Don't make your transformation any more difficult than it needs to be. Use the available free technology.

Using the current calorie counting technology will increase your precision dramatically thereby help you achieve better results. So let's talk about that.

The Dialed-In Approach (Technology Assisted)

These days there is quite a lot of technology available that makes the tasks of calorie counting and macronutrient tracking nearly effortless. I strongly encourage you to take advantage of one of the sophisticated web or phone applications available online to anyone. The best part is they cost nothing. I'll talk about specific tools at length in the next chapter, so bear with me while we dig into the macronutrients.

The Right Macro Ratios

In the previous chapter I discussed specific foods that you should be eating from the three macronutrient groups. Let's now talk about the right ratios of these foods. You already know your meal plan should be made up of intact whole foods from the three macro groups: (1) proteins, (2) fats and (3) carbohydrates. There are many schools of thought concerning the right macro ratios. There are those who advocate a high carb, low protein plan and those who believe in a high protein, high fat and low carb plan. Some nutritionists might also tell you that a balanced combination is best.

Personal experience has led me to one conclusion. Having tried them all, I strongly believe the optimum macronutrient ratio for shedding fat and building lean muscle is on the high protein and low carbohydrate end of the spectrum. I've found that a high protein and low carb approach best aids in muscle recovery and development. It also works best for losing fat and keeping it off. It's not just my own experience. A high protein and low carb nutrition plan has worked well for many people whose body compositions I've helped change. Both men and women of various ages and starting points have succeeded in achieving their goals. The high ratio of protein aids a great deal in muscle development, the calorie dense healthy fat is a source of fuel, and the low carbohydrate consumption promotes fat loss.

Start your body transformation with the following **macronutrient ratios: 45% protein, 35% fat and 20% carbohydrates.** You can always make adjustments if needed later on. If you find you're running out of energy, you can lower your protein 5% and raise your carbs 5%. If you're not satisfied with your muscle development you can raise your protein 5% and lower your fat 5%. We all have unique body chemistry so we'll respond differently to different sets of macro ratios. But begin with my recommended ratios and stick with them for at least the first 12 weeks, then reassess. You can make small changes periodically to your macro ratios as long as you stay within your total calories. The thing to remember is to stay the course and be patient. You may not notice changes day over day, but you *will* see significant results month to month.

Healthy Foods from Each Macronutrient Group

Probably the most difficult part of this entire program for most people will be to completely get off the processed carbohydrate train. Think of yourself as a recovering junkie and you've just started rehab. Cold turkey is the only way to go. Unfortunately, pasta from enriched flour, white bread and white rice are common dishes in popular food culture. You will be tested. You will at times be the odd man or odd woman out. You'll have to be strong of will. You'll have to break free from the herd and walk your own path. Stay the course and understand that there are certain foods you simply cannot – and should not – eat anymore.

However, I don't think it's realistic or even fair of anyone or me to just tell you "no," you have to stop eating these things. It's not reasonable to then leave it at that and expect the new behavior to last very long. In fairness you need healthy, good-tasting recommendations so that you know exactly what to eat. So here you go:

In order to trade that out of shape body for a fit lean body, you've got to trade processed carbohydrates for healthy alternatives such as whole grains and vegetables. Replace the pasta made from enriched white flour with whole grain pasta and a green vegetable like fresh asparagus. Replace white rice with whole grain brown rice and fresh broccoli. Replace white bread with whole grain bread. Get the picture? Have whole oatmeal with your breakfast instead of some sugar-laden cereal, whole grain rice with your lunch and some sweet potato with your dinner as your carbohydrate sources instead of pasta made from white flour. Swap the poison for medicine. Think of getting fit and lean as getting well. You're trading up, ultimately improving your quality of life.

The first week or two you may go through an adjustment period. You may not feel quite as satisfied (*ie,* stuffed) after meals. You'll also not feel the immediate gratification you once experienced albeit at a huge price. There's a reason that foods like pasta made from white flour and white breads are referred to as comfort foods. These foods do make you feel comfortable in as much as the insulin spike and subsequent blood sugar crash makes you feel like curling up on a coach and taking a nap. Too much comfort food and the struggle to stay awake afterwards can be overwhelming.

Like all deviations from the previous normal in life, you will quickly adapt. Your new nutrition plan will become your new normal and normal is going to feel great.

Lean Protein

For complete muscle recovery and optimal lean muscle development I recommend getting forty five percent of your calories from protein. Taking in this much **lean protein** everyday can be challenging. In fact, it can be downright difficult. In a perfect world, all your protein would come from whole food sources, but realistically that's a heck of a lot of food preparation. You may be asking, what does 45% of my daily calories from lean protein actually look like?

Let's say as an example that you're a 220-pound man whose target weight is 180 pounds. This means you should be eating 300 grams of protein per day. I strongly recommend eating six small meals a day as your body can only assimilate so much protein per serving. So doing the math, getting this amount of protein requires six 50-gram servings of protein every day. A practical solution is to make three to four of those protein sources from whole food sources like chicken breast, fish, lean red meat and egg whites. The other two or three protein servings can be a high quality protein powder. I'll discuss in greater detail what kind of protein powder as well as what other nutrition supplements are important in a later chapter on supplements.

Six serving of protein per day, one with each small meal, per day is both practical and reasonable. Bake some chicken breast in advance and package them up, so you can take 2 or 3 with you to work every day. Or hard-boil some eggs and eat the egg whites as a protein feed as one of your 6 small meals. Even in a situation where you have to eat out every meal of the day, there are almost always options available. For breakfast order an egg white omelet with extra egg whites (six egg whites is 22 grams of protein) and green vegetables. Add a side of oatmeal or whole grain toast for your carbohydrate. For lunch you can usually find a grilled chicken breast, salmon, beef or shrimp salad on the menu. For dinner order a lean protein (beef, chicken, or fish) with a green vegetable side and ask the waiter to ditch the starchy side of white flour pasta or white rice that's typically served, and replace it with a portion of green vegetables and/or a plain baked potato. If you're dining out and you're uncertain if the restaurant offers a lean protein on the menu, take along your own chicken breast or a ready to drink protein shake. If all else fails just skip your protein serving for a meal and fill up on salad, vegetables, complex carbohydrates and healthy fats. However, these days nearly any restaurant will make you something as a healthy lean protein if you request it. Just ask. Remember, you're in control of your health and fitness, not the restaurant.

Healthy Fats

Thirty five percent of your calories should come from **healthy fats**. Choose unsaturated fats over saturated fats. Fat is more calorie-dense than both protein and carbohydrates so less volume will yield more calories. For me, eating healthy fat is the most satisfying part of my nutrition plan. As a person who avoids eating processed foods, particularly refined carbohydrates and manufactured fats, I can attest to the fact that healthy fat has become my new comfort food. The satiated feeling we get from eating fats is a direct result of the calorie density of fat over protein and carbohydrates. Fat contains 9 calories per gram whereas protein and carbohydrates contain 4 calories per gram.

This makes fat not only more filling, but more satisfying as well. When I'm getting leaned out in a strictly controlled, calorie-restricted nutrition plan just a few months out from a physique contest, I crave fats. I savor them more than any other food. Natural peanut butter or the slightly healthier almond butter, with no added sugar of course, is the perfect healthy fat snack. Nut butter is a lifesaver really. Just 2 tablespoons of nut butter is 200 calories, most of which is healthy fat. Unsalted almonds are another easy snack to carry with you or keep in your desk at work. They are also calorie dense, high in healthy fat and very satisfying.

Avocados might just be Mother Nature's most nutritious healthy fat creation of all. Avocados are rich in unsaturated fat, vitamin B-6 and vitamin C, and they also contain about 15g of dietary fiber. Avocados satisfy hunger cravings and also taste great. I love the way they satisfy when I'm feeling like I've just got to eat something right now. These beautiful little green fruits are also very versatile in the kitchen. Yes, avocados are a fruit – but not one with a lot of sugar. They grow on trees and carry the plant's seed for reproduction. The avocado's ability to absorb and enhance other flavors is a wonderful culinary quality. As I mentioned in the previous chapter, fresh avocado on my egg white and chicken breast scramble in the morning soaks up my favorite hot sauce giving the meal a spicy kick. Sliced avocado on a bed of baby spinach soaks up balsamic vinegar and olive oil, creating a taste sensation. Be creative -- add them to your favorite lean protein or vegetable, and you just might stumble on an award winning new recipe.

Omega-3 and omega-6 fatty acids are considered essential because we can only obtain them through the food we eat. Our bodies do not have the ability to synthesize them. These healthy fats are found in olive oil, nut oils like flax seed and oily fishes such as salmon, mackerel and sardines. The great thing about oil rich cold-water fish is that you're able to get a protein serving and healthy fat serving all from the same source.

Olive oil is another great source of healthy fat. It's perfect for sautéing vegetables or a chicken breast. It can be used as cooking oil for scrambled egg whites or sautéed vegetables. Olive oil serves its purpose as a non-stick cooking oil as well as providing some of the healthy fat required in your nutrition plan. Now, when you're cooking with olive oil and other cooking oils such as canola oil or sunflower oil, be sure to remember their high calorie content (and log them into your calorie tracker). Use them sparingly because they're very calorie dense. One tablespoon will usually do for cooking vegetables or meats. You don't need a whole lot – just a little does the job and adds tremendous flavor.

Carbohydrates

Getting twenty percent of your calories from **carbohydrates** requires almost no effort. You'll find as you get into your nutrition plan that you spend most of your meal planning trying to *avoid* too many carbohydrates. Consider cultural meal norms the world over. Growing up in the Midwest United States, I was raised on meat and potatoes. A food staple in most Asian cultures is fish and rice. In much of Southern Europe some shape or form of pasta or bread is served with most every meal. Nearly every world culture's most common dishes combine a protein with a carbohydrate. What you'll soon discover is that sticking with this convention will put you way over on the amount of carbs and total calories you're allowed. This presents a real challenge whether you're ordering off a menu in a restaurant, attending a dinner party or dining at home with family. You'll need the dedication and willpower to break free from those cultural norms we've all been conditioned to follow since childhood. The solution is to stop eating breads and pastas. Replace such simple carbs with a reasonable portion of fiber-rich complex carbs, healthy fats and green vegetables.

Tag-Along Carbs

Ancillary carbohydrates, unintentional carbs, or "tag-along carbs," seem to be found in everything except protein sources. Tag-along carbs are in nearly everything we eat.

Let's draw a distinction between intentional carbs and tag-along carbs. I consider intentional carbs things we eat in order to fill our carbohydrate macronutrient requirement. Intentional carb choices should include whole oatmeal, whole-grain brown rice, whole grain bread, whole-grain pasta and sweet potatoes. Tag-along carbs are found in foods like green vegetable and nuts. We eat green vegetables like asparagus, broccoli and spinach primarily for the fiber and essential micronutrients (vitamins and minerals) they provide. You may be surprised at how fast these ancillary carbs add up. If, for example, your nutrition plan only allows for 150 grams of carbohydrates a day, you'll find that you max out your carbs easily. Without even adding intentional carbohydrate sources into your meal plan you'll probably reach your daily goal before dinner.

Common feedback I've gotten from those following my program is how difficult it is sometimes to get enough lean protein and healthy fat, whereas it's easy to fulfill their daily macro requirement of carbohydrates. Most folks aren't used to eating protein six times per day and there are limited sources of healthy fats available. This may be an adjustment that simply requires learning or training yourself to eat more protein and less carbohydrates. I realize that it's hard to break habits and tastes you've had since childhood, but it can be done.

Macronutrient Summary

Eating the right ratio of macronutrients is critical in changing your body composition. <u>Your nutrition plan should be made up of 45% lean protein, 35% healthy fat, and 20% complex carbohydrates.</u> The most accurate and efficient way to track both your calorie consumption and macronutrient ratios is by using a calorie counting app, utilizing the dialed in approach.

Eliminating refined carbohydrates, particularly sugar, is the single most important nutritional rule. Whole food complex carbs are good for you and are required, because your body needs carbohydrates for fuel. However, your body doesn't need them in the quantity you're probably accustomed to eating. You must eat them from the appropriate sources: lots of fresh vegetables and reasonable portions of whole grains. Even when limiting your carbohydrate sources specifically to these foods, you'll have to watch your intake closely as the calories and grams of carbohydrates add up fast.

Chapter 6

"There's no such thing as work-life balance. There are work-life choices, and you make them, and they have consequences."

- Jack Welch

Calorie Counting Made Easy

Your goal with the Get Fit, Lean Program is to change your body composition, which means losing fat and gaining lean muscle. In order to succeed, there are three critical things that you must do. First, you need to eat the right number of calories. This means you've got to count calories. Second, you've got to stay within your macronutrient ratios. Third, you need to eat the right foods within the macronutrient groups. Following these three fundamental nutrition rules is critical in achieving your fitness goals. Therefore, maintaining an accurate food diary is important.

Religiously maintaining an accurate food diary serves multiple purposes. To begin with, you'll be far less likely to cheat on your meal plan if you commit to logging every single thing that you eat. You'll avoid making bad food choices and instead make good food choices. Maintaining a record of everything you eat will also make it apparent how much the little things add up fast. You'll find that all the small snacks you might carelessly or mindlessly eat between meals will blow your calorie controlled nutrition plan out of the water.

Religiously logging every food item and staying within your daily calorie limits and macronutrient ratios will force you to stop and think twice about cheating on your nutrition plan. So when you track your food intake, don't lie or minimize your intake. Don't leave things out. Achieving your goals requires you to be honest about what you're eating so you can figure out if you're making any mistakes that can be corrected. After all, this is a learning process, and it takes time to get it right.

It's possible to track everything by hand using an actual logbook, however that would be extremely tedious and time consuming. This is where the online tools I mentioned last chapter come in very handy. Not only is using an online calorie (and macronutrient) counter more accurate, it's incredibly time efficient. Let modern technology do the otherwise tedious calculations and bookkeeping work for you. Plus, these tools also can give you information about a food ahead of time.

For example, when tempted by an unhealthy snack, or even just a snack that you may not be sure if it fits your nutrition plan or not, you can log it into the online counter first BEFORE you eat it to check its calorie and macronutrient make-up. This will let you see whether the extra calories and macronutrient profile would put you over your daily calorie limit or a macronutrient percentage. It will help you see whether you're getting too much of one macronutrient (like carbs). Or whether the calories will put you at a limit that prevents you from getting enough of one of the other important macronutrients you require, like protein.

Tracking everything you eat also makes meal planning for coming days much easier because you'll quickly become familiar with the calorie and macronutrient makeup of your regular meal choices. Last, and I think most important of all, is that when you keep track of all that you eat over time you will establish a personal calorie baseline.

Calorie Baseline

By a baseline, I mean that as time goes by you'll become more and more in touch with how your body responds to a certain number of calories. You'll become more dialed in. You will begin to feel in tune with your caloric needs as it relates to fat loss and lean muscle building. You will establish a calorie baseline whereby you'll know that if you eat X calories and burn Y calories then your weight will approach Z. I'll instruct you on how to begin and layout your initial 12-week nutrition plan. If you follow it faithfully, you'll get great results.

After the initial 12-week program you'll of course want to continue your fitness journey. You quite likely will need to tweak your nutrition plan a little as you continue to improve your body composition. Even though you'll have made amazing progress in your first 12 weeks, you may still want or need to add more lean muscle and lose additional fat. The baseline you establish will serve as a reference point that you can fall back on. This entire process is in part about you fine-tuning your machine. A high performance machine runs on a very precise fuel mix. Over time as you learn how your body reacts to subtle calorie changes and slight variations in your macronutrient ratios you'll become more and more dialed in. You will master your own body's nutritional and caloric requirements so you can make the best choices to get and keep you fit and lean.

Keeping a Meal Diary

Let's talk about how to keep a meal diary manually and also using one of the online/smartphone tools.

First we'll start with the simple "eyeball" method that I mentioned in Chapter 5. At best this is a close approximation, at worst this method is simply a wild guess. This calorie counting method is for the person who refuses to weigh or measure anything, just can't be bothered or doesn't have access to the modern technology that surrounds us. I strongly recommend using one of the free online calorie counting websites or smart phone apps to track it all.

Admittedly, I'm a Luddite at heart. Just a few years ago I fought tooth and nail the idea of adapting to this modern technology. But once I started using an online calorie and macronutrient counter, I never looked back. Doing so will help you in more ways than just keeping an accurate calorie and macronutrient count. If you are honest about logging everything you'll be far less likely to ever cheat on your nutrition plan. There is no hiding anything, so you'll be much more likely to make good food decisions.

Regardless of my advice, I'm sure there will be those who simply refuse to embrace modern technology. They will instead insist on estimating everything. So for them, here goes. Even for those of you who do faithfully commit to maintaining an online calorie counter please read this next section. Estimations will come in handy at times because the reality is that life is imperfect. You will at times find yourself in situations where you've got no choice but to estimate. This could be when dining out, a dinner party or traveling. You won't always have access to a scale or any practical way of measuring your food portions.

Estimating Protein Portions

Let's start with a common scenario, an average man trying to lose fat and build lean muscle. We'll assume your height is 5'11 and you weigh between 200 and 230 pounds. Your target weight is 175 to 185 pounds. I recommend a daily target calorie burn of 500 a day. Therefore, we'll also assume you're burning 500 calories a day doing cardio exercise.

First we need to outline your daily protein requirement. Your nutrition plan will consist of 250 to 300 grams of protein each day divided evenly between six meals a day, each meal giving you between 40 to 50 grams of protein. This is equivalent to eating six average-sized chicken breasts every day. Six chicken breasts every day would be pretty boring, huh? Instead, let's replace two of those with high quality protein shakes, one with an egg white scramble and one with a serving of fish or a lean red meat. So we have 2 meals with chicken breast, 2 meals with a protein shake, one with an egg scramble, and one with fish or read meat. That's not so boring is it? Heck, it's making me hungry! Now we're talking about the right fuel required to build some lean muscle.

Using the eyeball guide to approximate portion sizes, 4 oz of a lean protein is roughly the size of the palm of your hand. Therefore a 7-oz chicken breast, which is slightly less than double the size of the palm of your hand, is about 220 calories and 45 grams of protein. The following three portions contain very close to 50 grams of protein each: 6 oz of grilled fillet mignon, 7 oz of baked chicken breast and 8 oz of baked salmon. Eyeball the weight of these protein sources using the palm of your hand. Eat three to four of these every day then have a protein drink the other two to three meals and you've got your protein for the day. We'll cover what types of protein powders to look for as well as what other supplements are beneficial and how to choose the right ones in Chapter 13: Supplements.

Estimating Vegetables Portions

Estimating vegetable portions is more difficult than eyeballing lean proteins. Different vegetables have very different shapes and densities. Additionally, depending on the vegetable it may sometimes be easiest to measure it by weight whereas other times it may make more sense to measure it by volume. It might also be most practical to simply count average sized units of some food items. For example 20 average spears of asparagus is just over 100 calories and 20 grams of carbohydrates. The equivalent number of calories and grams of carbohydrates from broccoli is 3.5 cups. Your estimation guide for measuring vegetables is that 1 cup is about the same size as an average man's fist. The following table will help you approximate other common measurements.

Real World Measurement Approximations

1 teaspoon = size of one dice
2 tablespoons = size of a golf ball
1 cup = size of a man's fist
4 oz lean protein size of a man's palm
1 oz nuts fill the palm of a cupped hand
1 pound of fat = 3,500 calories (500 calories x 7 days)

As a general rule, your goal should be to eat 2 to 3 times the volume of green vegetables versus the volume of protein you're eating with at least two of your six meals every day. This is realistic and easy to do. Have a green salad with your lunch and a steamed or grilled green vegetable with your dinner. As I mentioned earlier, if you go overboard on anything in your nutrition plan, do it with green vegetables. Green vegetables are low in calories and chock full of vitamins and minerals.

Estimating Healthy Fats

Let's stick with the same scenario, a 5'11 guy who weighs between 200 and 230 pounds. He burns 500 calories a day doing cardio. He should be getting thirty percent of his calories from fat, which translates to about 90 to 100 grams of good (healthy) fat per day. Here is an example of a typical day's healthy fat consumption. One medium sized avocado is about 23 grams of fat. 2 oz of raw almonds contains 28 grams of fat. Three tablespoons of organic peanut butter adds in 25 more grams of fat. One tablespoon of extra virgin olive oil is an additional 14 grams of fat. All of these foods combined with the 2 and 3 grams of tag-along fats found in things like chicken breast and protein drinks easily get you to your required 100 grams of fat in a day. You could also eat an oily fish such as salmon. A 9 oz serving contains 21 grams of fat. If you choose the fish, you'll need to cut back on one of your other fat sources that day. That's where the advance meal planning that I mentioned earlier comes into play. By planning your meals in advance, you won't end up at the end of the day suddenly realizing you took in too much of one macronutrient or too little of another. It'll help you achieve that balance that will get you Fit and Lean.

Greater Accuracy for Greater Success: Apps and Websites

Use an online or smartphone app calorie counter! Is there any reason why you wouldn't use the most accurate, easiest and most efficient tools available? You'll be doing plenty of sweating in the gym so don't sweat trying to track your calories and macros by hand. *Use an online calorie counter!*

Calorie Counter Basics

There are several choices of free online or app based calorie counters available online. If you do a Google or App Store search for calorie counters, many will pop up. My favorite is MyFitnessPal.com (and in the interest of disclosure, I am receiving NO compensation from them for plugging this tool). But you're welcome to use the one that you think will work for you. Many of them sync with wearable bands like the Jawbone UPÒ band, Nike Fuelband,Ò and the like. That may play into your decision of which calorie counting app to use, if you are also using a wearable activity tracker.

At the heart of all the online calorie counters is a generic algorithm that will determine how many calories you should consume each day in order to reach a specific weight goal. You begin by first entering some personal details like your age along with your current weight. Then you enter your goal weight. For the purposes of the Get Fit, Lean program, your goal weight should be your target weight in 12 weeks' time. So if you're currently 175 pounds and want to be 150, then enter 150 as your goal weight.

The first thing the algorithm will calculate is your basal metabolic rate (BMR). Your BMR is the minimum number of calories required while at rest in order to live and maintain your current weight. The application will then ask you questions about your daily activity. It will ask the kind of work you do in order to determine how many calories you require above your BMR. The algorithm will take this into account to then determine your daily calorie in-take required to achieve your goal weight. If your goal is weight loss then you'll be burning more calories than you consume. You'll be in calorie deficit, which we discussed previously. This number of calories will typically be expressed as your daily calorie goal. This beginning calorie target does not include credit from cardio exercise (the app allows you to enter your daily cardio and cred-its those calories burned back to your daily total). We're concerned with *net calories,* so therefore you'll want it to add the calories burned doing cardio as a calorie credit. This is a great incentive to do your daily cardio because you're allowed to consume those additional calories burned (I'll discuss this in more detail shortly).

Setting Up Your Macronutrient Ratios

Although your total calories are important, making sure the counter is calculating and tracking your macronutrient ratios is extremely important. Your daily intake of the right ratios of proteins, carbs, and fats is a crucial to changing your body composition. However, you'll have to manually set your macronutrient ratios, because typically the default ratios in the calorie counting apps are designed for the average person who only wants to lose weight. I believe they are far too low in protein and far too high in carbohydrates for someone like you whose goal is to change your body composition by losing fat and gaining lean muscle rather than simply losing scale weight. Consider yourself an athlete. Even if you've never thought of yourself this way before, do so now because you're now taking the first step in becoming an athlete. The default macro settings will be far too many carbohydrates and far too little protein for losing fat and gaining lean muscle like you'll be doing. Therefore, you'll have to manually set your macronutrient ratios as a percentage of your total calories to reflect the optimum targets of the Get Fit, Lean program. **I recommend starting with 45% protein, 35% fat and 20% carbohydrates.**

Setting Up Your Meal Plan Diary and Nutrition Components

MyFitnessPal also allows you to customize your meal plan entry screen. I recommend that you set up your meal plan diary for six meals per day – basically you'll be consuming three meals a day with three snacks added in, so it's easiest to track as six separate meals a day. It's also much easier to spread your food intake throughout the day.

MyFitnessPal.com also allows you to track six different components of nutrition. This means that the app allows you to set up six columns, each with its own header, across your food diary page. This allows you to track six different components of your meal plan. *Set up these columns first with the following:*

Total Calories

Protein

Carbohydrates

Fat

The remaining two nutrients I advise you to track are:

Sugar

Sodium

Tracking sugar is important because sugar is the one food component that you are trying as hard as possible to minimize. If you follow my program correctly you will be trying your best to completely eliminate refined carbohydrates, specifically sugar and refined flour, from your meal plan. Your daily total sugar consumption should be approaching only 20 to 30 grams per day maximum. Zero sugar would be ideal, but is not realistic as there are naturally occurring sugars in many of the foods you'll be eating. You'll find that many food items like sweet potatoes or peanut butter for example contain a few grams of sugar. You'll also see that although they are a good source of fiber and are vitamin-loaded, most fruits contain significant amounts of sugar. As I mentioned previously, until you reach your weight goal, it's best to avoid eating fruit. If you are craving fruit, eat a small portion of a fruit that is low on the glycemic index. Two or three ounces of cherries, blueberries, blackberries or strawberries are good choices.

Additionally, keep your sodium intake within your daily limit. Remember, sodium is salt. Tracking and limiting your salt intake is important for a couple of good reasons. First, people prone to high blood pressure should be monitoring their salt intake anyway. Second, too much salt will make you retain water, because your body is always trying to achieve equilibrium. The natural occurring water in our bodies is basically salt water. Too much salt in our food makes us retain extra water until we're able to flush it out with more water and return it to a healthy equilibrium. People who consume too much salt are subsequently and needlessly carrying around extra water weight. They are perpetually bloated.

There's actually another good reason to monitor your sodium intake. If you notice that you are frequently exceeding your targeted daily sodium intake, it's a very good indicator that you're eating some unhealthy processed food-like products – most likely something packaged in a box or a can that contains salt as a preservative or flavor additive. The two primary functions of added salt in food packaging are improving or enhancing flavor and extending shelf life. Salt is a great preservative. It's not uncommon for people who eat pre-packaged processed foods and live primarily on fast foods to get *several hundred* times the amount of sodium they actually require for good health. Do you think there are negative health consequences from chronic sodium over loading? You bet there are. So if you follow the Get Fit, Lean program, most of your meal plan should come from fresh intact whole foods, therefore you won't have a sodium problem. Track your sodium intake and this will quickly become apparent.

Cardio Calorie Credits

Let's talk for a bit about the credited calories I mentioned earlier. The total calories available for you to eat on a daily basis are net calories, not gross calories. This means that the calories you burn doing cardio exercise counts as a credit towards your total calorie intake. If you do more cardio, you get to eat more - so how's *that* for motivation to do your cardio? There's an input for calories burned doing cardio exercise on your meal plan diary.

Here's the rub. Beware of what the machines at your gym say you've burned. In my years of experience trying out as many different cardio machines as I can, I've found that most will greatly exaggerate your total calories burned. My speculative explanation is that because the major cardio equipment manufacturers want you to choose *their* machine over their competitor's cardio machine, calories burned outputs tend to be very generous. They know that people will more likely choose and then use the machines with the greatest calories burned output. If this sounds too much like conspiracy theory to you then please test my hypothesis. Wear a good quality heart rate monitor while using a piece of cardio equipment and compare results. The heart rate monitor manufacturers don't have any vested interest in exaggerating your calories burned. They are simply computing an accurate as possible calorie burn output. If you don't want to invest in a heart rate monitor then do what I do. Correct for the cardio machine exaggeration by entering just two thirds of whatever the calories burned output displays. If you spend forty-five minutes on an elliptical machine and the calories burned output is 800 calories then enter 533 (2/3 of 800) in your food diary app or website. I've tested this using a good heart rate monitor against several different machines and 2/3 is usually very close to the actual calories burned.

Your Progress and Food Diary History

Record your weight daily. Weigh yourself every morning and enter it in your online calorie counter. Weigh yourself first thing in the morning as soon as you get out of bed before you've had anything to eat or drink. Although the mirror will tell the real story, your scale weight is also a pretty good metric of your progress. Your weight may not change much while your body composition is changing dramatically. It depends on how much actual body fat you started with. Recording and entering body measurements is also of what the machines at your gym say you've burned. MyFitnessPal allows for this as well. Take a weekly, bi-weekly, or a monthly measurement of your arms, chest, waist, hips and any other body part that you'd like to improve. If you work out at a health club, another metric you can have one of the staff help you with is to track your body fat % using the caliper method. Although this isn't the most accurate method, having someone checking your skinfold fat thickness on a weekly basis can be very motivating and can help reinforce your progress, or it can tell you if you're not making progress, which means you need to look at what you're doing and see what's off. The bottom line is, monitoring your progress will provide positive reinforcement that will help you stay on track as you see yourself making real changes, or alert you if you need to make adjustments to your meal plan or activity level.

Another benefit of maintaining your online meal diary, weight and periodic measurements is that you'll be establishing a personal history. Over time, after collecting enough data points, you'll be able to chart your progress as well as go back and see how well you are staying on course. I've found that this helps me a great deal because I'm able to identify trends. You will begin to see the correlation of staying true to the program and your resulting weight changes. You'll also see how small adjustments yield significant results over time. At some point you may need to tweak your plan a bit. Because you've recorded your history, you'll know the calorie adjustment or exercise modification that you need to take your weight up or down.

Weight Loss Is *NOT* a Straight Line Function

First, for consistency, I recommend weighing yourself first thing every morning before you've had anything to eat or drink. There is an extremely important point about weight loss that you need to understand for your own motivation and sanity. *Your weight loss will not occur in a continuous straight line.* What is important is that over time, the trend is moving in the right direction. Picture what the daily bar chart of a company's stock price typically looks like. There are small daily fluctuations, but the long-term trend is usually moving either up or down. Typically, you will see small daily fluctuations both up and down, as well as some days when your weight doesn't change at all. Don't get discouraged when you see this happening; it's completely normal and you should expect it. There are a couple good explanations why this happens.

First, when viewed through an evolutionary lens, this is a great example of our highly tuned survival mechanism at work. When you put yourself in calorie deficit, your body will initially react by hanging onto its fat stores. You are confronting your basic biological drive to eat and to defend against weight loss.[48] The simple act of eating fewer calories than you burn combined with some cardio exercise will ring survival mode alarm bells in your brain. Fewer calories and more exercise will be interpreted as a crisis situation at first. Your body will most likely fight back and stubbornly resist giving up its energy reserves: your fat stores. This effect is temporary and usually only lasts a few days or a few weeks at the most – so stick with it. After a short amount of time your body will adapt to your new food intake and exercise regimen and you'll begin losing weight again. What typically happens is this: you'll weigh the same for several days in a row with little or no change, and then one morning you get on the scale and are surprised to find that you've dropped two pounds.

Second, daily weight fluctuations are significantly influenced by your salt intake, which we just discussed, emphasizing the need to monitor and manage sodium. Water is heavy. If you've taken in more sodium than usual the previous day, your weight can easily jump up a pound or two simply because you're temporarily holding a little extra water to compensate for the unusual salt consumption. We humans are made of 70% (salt) water and our bodies are continually trying to achieve a salt equilibrium, so a small variation in salt can lead to significant water retention. Maintain a low to normal sodium nutrition plan, and those extra pounds will disappear as fast as they appeared.

Daily weight fluctuations are normal. Don't let the small variations discourage you, and focus on the long-term trend making sure it's heading in the right direction over time. It's much like investing in the stock market - except you want this trend to go down. The same financial market adage applies; the trend is your friend. If the trend begins going the wrong way, then you'll have to make some adjustment by pulling one or both of the available levers. You'll either have to reduce your calorie intake by consuming less or increase the calories you burn by doing a little more cardio exercise.

Tweaking the Macronutrient Ratios

We've covered a lot in this chapter and it's important to understand that tracking total calories is important but it's equally important to track your macronutrient ratios. Optimizing your mix of protein, fat and carbs is critical in order to change your body composition. You may very well be asking how this guy knows that a macro mix of 45% protein, 35% fat and 20% carbs is right for me. Fair enough question.

Everyone has unique body chemistry, and so everyone will react a little differently to different ratios of macronutrients. Over the years I've tried several different ratios of macros and have settled on the mix that I'm advising you to start with in my Get Fit Lean program. I don't believe my recommended macro ratios to be extreme in any one direction. My request to you is this: stick with it for at least a month and see how much your body reacts. Then assess how you are feeling and progressing. I'm betting that you'll have seen enough results that you'll agree these are good baseline macronutrient ratios.

Combining sound macronutrient management wit with calorie control and exercise, you *will* get results and you *will* achieve your weight goal. If, after the first month you're feeling a severe lack of energy, bump up the carbs to 25% and lower the protein to 40%. If you feel like after 12 weeks that you've got plenty of energy and you'd like to accelerate your fat loss while you build more muscle, then you can bump up the protein to 50% and lower the carbs to 15%. It's your body and only you will know how you feel. This is part of the process of getting dialed in, self-discovery, and understanding your own body. A key aspect of the Get Fit, Lean program is that after the first 12 weeks you will have established a net calorie baseline. You will know how your body responds to X amount of calories in, and Y amount of calories burned. You'll also begin to get a feel for how your body responds to a given ratio of macronutrients. The total calories you need to consume will be easiest to define. Put yourself in calorie deficit mode and you'll lose weight. But when it comes to the ratio of macros, there will likely be some trial and error involved. This is normal and should be expected.

It's a Calorie Optimization Problem

For you analytically inclined people who prefer to frame your transformation in quantitative terms, think of this entire process as one big optimization problem. In order to lose net weight (fat) you need to put yourself in calorie deficit. In order to change your body composition (replace fat with lean muscle) you need to eat the right ratio of macronutrients. One pound of fat is 3,500 calories, so if you burn 500 calories a day more than you consume you should lose one pound a week (500 x 7 = 3,500). For optimal results, you should make the most efficient use of your available calories each day. Your macro calorie ratios of 45% protein, 35% fat and 20% carbs should come from the highest quality sources possible. Think of your nutrition plan in terms of maximizing your calorie input.

Chapter 7

"Failing to plan is planning to fail."

- Benjamin Franklin

Sample Meal Plans

You now know what to eat. Eat fresh intact whole foods from the three macronutrient groups. The online calorie counter you've chosen will calculate the total number of daily calories you're allowed in order to reach your goal weight. You will have manually set your macronutrient ratios to 45% protein, 35% fat and 20% carbs. You're ready to start tracking your nutrition plan.

The next few pages are sample meal diaries based on the foods I like best. Everyone has different tastes, so you can choose mine and tweak it, or substitute other foods that you like. I've also included lists of good food recommendations for every macronutrient group at the end of this chapter so you can switch things up and have some variety in your meals. As long as the foods you pick meet our previously discussed criteria of being fresh, intact whole foods and adhering to the calorie and macronutrient profiles, swapping one for another is perfectly fine. If you don't like chicken, swap it for fish or a steak. If you don't like asparagus, swap it for spinach or broccoli. Swap a baked russet potato for a sweet potato, or whole grain bread for oatmeal. There are plenty of options, and picking the foods you like and enjoy eating (that fit our criteria) will increase your chance of success. Staying on the plan is what is most important.

Your starting point and your target goal weight will determine how many total calories you're allowed. Try to divide your calories evenly throughout the day's meals. This will take a bit of trial and error on your part. It may seem a bit cumbersome at first, but it no time at all you'll be familiar with the portion sizes of your favorite foods that work for each meal. We're all creatures of habit and tend to eat most of the same foods day to day. In fact, I eat pretty much the same meals every day for breakfast and lunch. It might sound boring, but I'm busy and it works for me. I do try and eat a different meal for my sit down dinner every evening. After a few years of using MyFitnessPal I still log a new food into the system to check its calorie and macronutrient totals before eating it, to make sure I know exactly what portion size fits into my nutrition plan. You'll be doing this either online, on your desktop computer or on a mobile connected device, and it will be important that you are willing to experiment. If you are over or under on calories or macros in a certain day, then make adjustments for the next day by tweaking the portion sizes until they fit your plan. If you're uncertain about a new food's nutrient profile, then log it into the program and look at its profile before you eat it. You can't undo it if you err on eating too large of a portion. Well, not gracefully anyway. It's no fun to eat something, log it in, and THEN realize you just consumed 80% of your day's carbohydrates and you have to figure out what to eat the rest of the day that won't put you over your carb limit. So check it before you eat it!

Another useful tip is to plan your meals for the entire day using the calorie counter app – ideally the day before, or even try to plan a week at a time, if you can do that. After you become familiar with the correct portion size of your most frequently eaten foods, you can start logging meal by meal. If you try and log meals after the fact, it's too easy to go over on calories or macronutrients. So plan out your meals ahead of time, and take the potential for "oh no, I slipped up and ate too much of X" out of the equation.

In addition to planning your meals in advance, I highly recommend planning your cardio exercise in advance. Remember, the calories you burn doing cardio is a credit towards the total calories that you're allowed to consume every day. "Net calories" consumed is what you are tracking. If you plan to burn 350 calories tomorrow running on the treadmill for 30 minutes then add that into your meal diary and plan your calorie consumption accordingly. An added benefit of planning your cardio in advance is that you're much more likely to follow through and do the exercise. Since you've already accounted for the calories in your meal plan, you are committed.

My last tip is to persuade a friend, partner, husband, wife or family member to start using the online calorie counter with you. The calorie counting app may seem a bit like just another social media platform that you don't have time for, but it's not. This tool can help motivate you and help you achieve your goals through its ability to let other people see your progress and your meal plans. And although you can send messages to your MyFitnessPal "friends," the most useful benefit of having friends using the same calorie counting app is that it keeps you honest and gives you a support person or group. You can check out one another's meal plans, helping each other stay on track. In addition to checking up on each other, this feature is also great for getting food ideas from your friends. Most importantly you're more likely to religiously log your meals and be honest knowing that your friends can view your diary. If you had dinner with them and they can see what you logged, they'll know if you left something out of your diary. So look at this feature as setting up a support group. Encouragement from your MyFitnessPal friends will help you succeed in achieving your goals.

The following examples are what a meal diary might look like. The meals chosen below are typical foods from my diary. The first example is that of a person with total allowed calories before cardio of 2,300 and in the second example the person's total allowed calories before cardio is 1,700. Calories are expressed in actual calories. All other macronutrient values are expressed in grams.

Meal Plan Example #1 (2300 calorie plan)

Meal #1	Calories	Protein	Carbs	Fat	Sugar	Sodium
Oatmeal, Quick Cooking						
.5 cup	154	5	27	3	0	3
Whey Protein						
2 Scoops	170	36	3	2	2	80
Organic Peanut Butter						
2 tbsp	200	8	6	17	2	85
Totals	**524**	**49**	**36**	**22**	**4**	**168**
Meal #2						
Egg Whites Only						
6	102	22	1	0	0	330
Chicken Breast, diced						
3 oz	141	26	0	3	0	63
Whole Grain Tortillas						
1	90	5	14	1	0	200
Avocado, Raw						
0.5	161	2	9	15	1	7
Totals	**494**	**55**	**24**	**19**	**1**	**600**
Meal #3						
Whey Protein						
2 Scoops	170	36	3	2	2	80
Totals	**170**	**36**	**3**	**2**	**2**	**80**
Meal #4						
Chicken Breast						
5 oz	235	44	0	5	0	105
Whole Grain Tortilla						
1	90	5	14	1	0	200
Almonds, Unsalted						
1 oz	164	6	6	15	1	0
Totals	**489**	**55**	**20**	**21**	**1**	**305**
Meal #5						
Fillet Mignon (Grilled)						
5 oz	255	39	0	10	0	85
Sweet Potato, Baked						
4 oz	104	2	24	0	10	0
Asparagus, Grilled						
20 spears	100	8	16	0	0	12
Olive Oil, Extra Virgin						
0.5 tbsp	60	0	0	7	0	0
Totals	**519**	**49**	**40**	**17**	**10**	**97**
Meal #6						
Casein Protein						
2 scoops, 64 g	240	48	8	2	0	110
Organic Peanut Butter						
2 tbsp	200	8	6	17	2	85
Totals	**440**	**56**	**14**	**19**	**2**	**195**
Totals	**2636**	**300**	**137**	**100**	**20**	**1445**
Your Daily Goal	2650	298	133	103	59	2500
Remaining	14	-2	-5	3	39	1055
	Calories	**Protein**	**Carbs**	**Fat**	**Sugar**	**Sodium**

*You've earned 350 extra calories from exercise today

Meal Plan Example #2 (1700 calorie plan)

Meal #1	Calories	Protein	Carbs	Fat	Sugar	Sodium
Multi Grain Bread						
1 slice	90	5	15	1	2	180
Whey Protein						
1 Scoop	85	18	2	1	1	40
Organic Peanut Butter						
2 tbsp	200	8	6	17	2	85
Totals	**375**	**31**	**23**	**19**	**5**	**305**
Meal #2						
Egg Whites Only						
6	102	22	1	0	0	330
Multi Grain Bread						
1 slice	90	5	15	1	2	180
Avocado, Raw						
0.50	161	2	9	15	1	7
Totals	**353**	**29**	**25**	**16**	**3**	**517**
Meal #3						
Whey Protein						
2 Scoop	170	36	2	1	1	40
Totals	**170**	**36**	**2**	**1**	**1**	**40**
Meal #4						
Chicken Breast						
4 oz	141	26	0	3	0	63
Multi Grain Bread						
1 slice	90	5	17	0	1	180
Almonds, Unsalted						
1 oz	164	6	6	15	1	0
Totals	**395**	**37**	**23**	**18**	**2**	**243**
Meal #5						
Salmon (Grilled)						
4 oz	232	25	0	14	0	365
Baked Potato						
3 oz	82	2	18	0	2	13
Spinach						
4 cups	28	4	4	0	1	96
Totals	**342**	**31**	**22**	**14**	**3**	**474**
Meal #6						
Casein Protein						
1 scoops, 32 g	240	48	8	2	0	55
Organic Peanut Butter						
2 tbsp	200	8	6	17	2	85
Totals	**440**	**56**	**14**	**19**	**2**	**140**
Totals	**2075**	**220**	**109**	**87**	**16**	**1719**
Your Daily Goal	2050	231	103	80	36	1525
Remaining	-25	11	-7	-7	20	-194
	Calories	**Protein**	**Carbs**	**Fat**	**Sugar**	**Sodium**

*You've earned 350 extra calories from exercise today

Again, notice that the total calorie goal for Meal Plan #1 was 2650 after adding in the cardio credit. This number was originally 2300 before the cardio exercise credit of 350 calories burned was logged. In Meal Plan #2 the total calories available to eat were 1700 before the cardio credit of 350 calories burned was added. This shows you how doing your cardio helps give you additional calorie credits so you can eat a little more that day. Pretty cool, huh?

Also, note that in both examples the calorie goal and macronutrient goals were not reached perfectly. That's ok. Try to get as close as you can, but understand that it's difficult to hit the numbers dead on.

Your long-term success depends a great deal on you choosing healthy foods that you enjoy eating. Read nutrition labels. Cook with zero calorie spices and try to make foods taste interesting. Eat as little sugar as you can. With a little effort and creativity in the kitchen, healthy foods can certainly be delicious. Choose foods that you like and be sure that they fit into your nutrition plan before you start eating. If you enjoy what you're eating, you'll greatly improve your chances of success.

How to Deal with Long Days at the Office and Traveling

You may very well be thinking, "If I had a fully stocked kitchen in my office at my disposal, this eating right thing sure would be a lot easier." You're absolutely right. But in reality, most of us with normal jobs and offices don't have this luxury, so how do you handle eating right in the real world? The answer is simple: plan your meals at least a day in advance, and learn to prepare food in portions that will cover multiple meals. In addition, plan your meals and bring them along wherever you go. Investing in a small portable cooler and some freezer packs is something you can do in order to have a traveling "mini-fridge" for your meals that you can take almost anywhere – even your office or cubicle at work.

Chicken breasts, my go-to protein source, are something I cook 8 to 12 at a time. Just sprinkle on a little seasoning salt or your favorite low-salt dry rub, and they taste great. Bag them up and throw them in the refrigerator or freezer. I can easily go through 1 to 2 pounds of chicken breast a day, so cooking them in bulk makes a lot of sense. And they can be the protein staple in most meals. Take an 8 ounce chicken breast, an ounce of almonds, and a sweet potato or a whole grain tortilla and you've got a great meal on the go consisting all three macronutrients.

Unless you're lucky enough to have a gourmet cafeteria in your office building you're probably going to have to take a few meals to work every day. Long days of traveling will also require a few meals in hand. Chicken breast, almonds, peanut butter, brown rice, whole grain bread and baked sweet potatoes are easy foods to bring along in your small cooler. You can't rely on fast food restaurants around your office building or the airport food court for your meals. You're going to have to get used to the idea of preparing on-the-go meals in advance if you want to succeed.

List of *Healthy* Food Recommendations by Macronutrient Group

Proteins
- Egg whites
- Chicken & turkey breast
- White fish (halibut & cod)
- Oily fish (salmon, mackerel, and sardines)
- Lean beef
- Bison
- Shrimp
- Lobster
- Low-fat cottage cheese
- Plain Greek yogurt (no sugar added)
- Wild game meat (venison, antelope, pheasant, and quail)

Fats
- Avocado
- Nuts (almonds & walnuts)

- Peanut, almond, and other nut butters
- Oily fish (salmon, mackerel, and sardines)
- Olives and olive oil
- Flax oil
- Krill oil

Carbohydrates
- Sweet potatoes
- White and red potatoes (in moderation)
- Whole grain brown rice
- Squash
- Quinoa
- Whole grain oatmeal
- Whole grain pasta
- Whole grain bread
- Legumes (black beans, chick peas)
- Green vegetables (all)
- Fresh fruit (limited amounts until you reach your weight goal)

List of *Unhealthy* Foods to Avoid

Sugar, High Fructose Corn Syrup, and Flour (Refined Carbs)
- Soft drinks, cola, soda, sweet teas, energy drinks (all beverages with added sugar)
- White bread, brown bread, wheat bread (only eat bread that is made from *whole grains*)
- Bagels
- Cake, doughnuts, brownies, croissants, and cookies
- Tortillas (made from flour or corn)
- Pasta (unless made from *whole grains*)
- Yogurt (sweetened yogurt, plain Greek is good)

- Ketchup and BBQ Sauce
- Cereals (especially sugared children's breakfast cereal)
- Movie theater popcorn
- Coffee drinks, the carb-infused varieties

Trans Fat
- Fast foods, French fries are especially bad
- Packaged cookies
- Cake frosting
- Pancakes
- Microwave popcorn
- Frozen meals

MSG (Monosodium Glutamate) Laden Foods
- Bottled salad dressings
- Fried foods
- Potato chips

Sodium Overloaded Foods
- Packaged/deli lunch meats
- Salty snacks like pretzels
- Pizza
- Processed cheese

Chapter 8

"My motto was always to keep swinging. Whether I was in a slump or feeling badly or having trouble off the field, the only thing to do was keep swinging."

- Hank Aaron (MLB's True Home Run King)

Cardio Training

Run, bike, swim, snow ski, kick box, hop on an elliptical machine, climb on a stair machine or run on a treadmill. It doesn't matter what type of cardiovascular exercise you choose. What is important is that you're getting your blood pumping, working up a good sweat and most of all you are getting your heart rate up. If you get your heart rate up and sweat, chances are you're burning a lot of calories.

Cardiovascular (cardio) training is all about getting your heart rate up. Boosting your heart rate increases your metabolic rate, which causes your body to burn a lot of calories during cardio exercise. There's a significant residual benefit as well. Cardio exercise tends to keep your metabolism running a little higher than it would otherwise for hours or even days after each session.[49] The benefit of this is an obvious one. In addition to burning calories while doing the cardio exercise itself you'll be burning more calories in between your cardio sessions, even while at rest. So it's critical that you engage in regular cardio exercise as part of the Get Fit, Lean program. Cardio is one of the three key components of the program. In this chapter, I'll instruct you on finding the right target heart rate, tracking calories burned, and using cardio exercise to burn fat.

Hit Your Target Heart Rate

The term "target heart rate" means the optimal heart rate for burning calories during cardio exercise. When you are doing cardio at a pace that puts your heart rate consistently in your target heart rate range, you will be turning yourself into a fat burning machine.

Target heart rate varies somewhat depending on age and a few other factors. What then should YOUR target heart rate be? First of all, let's assume you're in good health and able to safely exercise. If you've any possible health concerns or you've not had a comprehensive physical exam for some time, then you should go see a doctor before doing any kind of intense exercise. You should not start any kind of nutrition or exercise plan without first consulting with your doctor. This program assumes that you have done so.

Second, it depends on how many calories you want/need to burn and how much time you have to exercise? You can burn as many calories doing 12 minutes of intense 1-minute intervals of sprinting and jogging as you can by doing a 45-minute steady state (constant speed) run. It's also important to find exercises that you like and are comfortable doing. I recommend that you have a calorie burn goal. You can calculate your calories burned during cardio exercise using either a good quality heart rate monitor or a cardio exercise machine at your gym. Both will display the number of calories burned as outputs. Just remember, as I mentioned before, if you rely on your gym's machines, reduce the displayed calorie burn to 2/3 since they are almost always inflated to some degree.

Although we all have different tolerances for physical stress and activity, the following table is a good guide for where your target heart rate should be.

Target Heart Rate/Fat Burning Zone

220 – (your age) = X (maximum present heart rate)

X * .75 = lower limit

X * .85 + upper limit

Example: You are 35 years old

220 – 35 = 185

185 * .75 = 138.75 (lower heart rate)

185 * .85 = 157.25 (upper heart rate)

So what this example shows is that for a 35 year old, your heart rate should be between 138.75 and 157.25 (or rounded to 139-157) beats per minute (bpm). That's where your body will be optimally burning fat and calories. So you need to be performing your cardio exercise at an intensity level that gets your heart rate between 139 and 157 bpm.

Keeping Your Cardio Fresh

As you follow my program, you'll be spending more time doing cardio than you will weight training. Using a variety of different fitness center machines or outdoor cardio exercises will keep your routine from becoming, well, a routine. Utilizing different machines or exercises on different days keeps it a bit more interesting and changes up the muscles you are working during your cardio training.

Many people find cardio training boring, or at least difficult to focus on for 30 to 45 minutes. Here's a tip: I keep it interesting by changing machines or exercises frequently and either listening to music or watching the TV monitors lined up in front of the cardio training area (if I'm doing cardio inside). I sometimes wonder if I'd be able to get through my cardio at all without ESPN SportsCenter to take my mind off the fact that my heart rate is at 145 bpm and I'm drenched in sweat.

I also know people who can't get through their run or bike ride without a good, motivational music mix. Take the time to set up some gym mixes on your music player and you can then set it to shuffle.

Remember, your goal when doing your cardio is to get your heart rate up and burn calories. You burn calories most effectively by speeding up your metabolism. You speed your metabolic rate by increasing your heart rate. With the right resistance, speed and intensity you can accomplish this on a treadmill, stair machine, elliptical machine, stationary bike, swimming laps in a pool, or get outside and run, bike, swim, roller blade or whatever gets your heart rate up. Choose the machines and methods that you are most comfortable with, and be sure to keep it fresh by doing different things on different days.

My Favorite Cardio Machines

Cardio machine engineering, like everything else in our modern world, continues to improve as technology advances. One of my favorite cardio machines is the Open Stride Adaptive Motion Trainer made by the PrecorÒ Company. Precor's AMTÒ machine gives you the feel of a natural movement like running but without the impact. Knees, back, and other parts of our frame take quite a bit of pounding when running on a hard surface. There is no impact using the AMT or other elliptical machines. I'm able to get my heart rate to 145 bpm and maintain that for 30 to 60 minutes depending on my cardio goal that day. I believe, for the sake of longevity, low to no impact machines are the best choice. Other low impact cardio choices are step/stair machines, elliptical machines and stationary bikes.

Calorie Deficit

In order to lose weight by losing body fat you've got to put yourself in calorie deficit. I'm sure you remember the simple thermal dynamics formula we discussed earlier: burn more calories than you consume, and you'll lose weight. Cardio training is a large part of the "burn more calories" half of the equation. By now I hope you're committed to using an online calorie counter to keep track of the calories and macronutrients you eat (the "calories consumed" part of the equation). Doing so will make this entire process much easier than estimating portion sizes and trying to keep an accurate calorie count by hand. Greater accuracy will lead to greater success.

This plays into the benefit I mentioned when discussing the calorie counting apps: cardio training creates a calorie credit that then allows you to eat more. The actual cardio training you do is a credit towards the calories you get to eat that day. When we talk about calorie intake for the day, we're talking about net calories. For example, if your nutrition plan target is 2300 calories per day to get you to your goal weight, and you burn 350 calories doing 30 minutes of cardio training that day, then you get to eat a total of 2650 total calories that day. This may not seem like much, but once you get going and are true to your calorie controlled meal plan, those extra 350 calories will seem like a small feast. Believe me, the additional calories you get to consume will be especially rewarding at the end of a day if you're hungry and all that is keeping you loyal to the program is sheer will power.

Heart Rate Monitors and Tracking Cardio Calories Burned

As I've probably made clear by now, I was once a Luddite or maybe at best a slow adaptor of technology. Even after years of encouragement by various spin bike instructors, competitive endurance athlete friends and personal trainer friends, I resisted buying a heart rate monitor. I thought to myself, I work hard. I sweat. It's working. I'm getting results. Why do I need to measure my heart rate? Well, my attitude about that was wrong.

As I became more and more precise in tracking my total calorie consumption, macronutrient ratios, and calories burned, I realized that I was merely estimating the inputs. If you're going to do something, why not do it right? You're investing a lot of both time and energy into transforming yourself so why not make the most of it? Why approximate anything by guessing when you don't have to? Why not dial it all in as precisely as you can? Investing in a heart rate monitor helps you be more precise and is money well spent. It allows you to know exactly how many calories you've burned every time you do any cardio exercise. If the cardio you choose is something outside like running or biking, you'll have no accurate way of knowing how many calories you burn. Therefore, I strongly recommend you remove the guesswork and get yourself dialed in.

A heart rate monitor monitors two important variables that are important for maximum calorie and fat burning. First, you'll be able to achieve and stay in your fat burning target heart rate zone, because you'll have a real time display of your heart rate while you're exercising. Second, you'll know exactly how many calories you've burned and can input this in your calorie counter as a credit towards your food consumption.

Depending on the exercise you choose for your cardio training, and if you do most of your training in a gym or fitness center, you don't necessarily *have* to buy a heart rate monitor. Most cardio machines have built-in heart rate monitors. There are sensors built into the handgrips that monitor your heart rate in real time. When you grip the sensors the machine reads your pulse. Based on other personal input data the machine calculates your total calories burned based on your heart rate.

As I've already mentioned, the thing to remember is that the total calories burned output on most cardio exercise machines is very generous. My experience has been that whether it's a treadmill, elliptical trainer, stair machine or whatever piece of cardio equipment I choose, gym cardio machines systematically output significantly more calories than the actual number of calories I burned. Typically, when you first get on one of these machines it will ask you to input your personal information. The cardio machine's onboard computer has a built-in algorithm that calculates the total calories you burn based on variables such as weight, age, time spent exercising and your actual (or estimated) heart rate while exercising.

Why am I so critical of these machines and sure that they aren't completely accurate? Because I've tested the accuracy of many cardio machines by wearing a heart rate monitor while using the machine, and then compared the outputs. I've nearly always gotten very different results. Depending on the manufacturer, the true number of calories burned on my heart rate monitor is significantly less (on average only about two thirds) than the machine output. The actual calories burned are on average about two thirds of what the machine display outputs. Ask any serious cardio junkie, fitness enthusiast or an experienced personal trainer at your gym if they've worn a heart rate monitor. If they've also tested their cardio machines accuracy, and if they're honest, they'll tell you the same thing.

Don't worry. This small distortion is not going to derail your cardio training in the least. There are a couple of easy enough solutions. First, buy and wear a good quality heart rate monitor as I have recommended. You can customize it with your personal details and most importantly, you can trust the calories burned output. Heart rate monitors are designed for serious competitive athletes such as triathletes and distance runners, so the manufacturers' only vested interest is accuracy. Heart rate monitor manufacturers are in competition with one another to build the most reliable and accurate equipment, not the one that outputs the greatest calories burned number.

If you don't want to buy a heart rate monitor or can't afford one right now, then use the next best solution. Use the machines' output and then compensate for the cardio machine's exaggerated calorie burn by recording just two thirds of whatever the cardio machine outputs. This is of course an approximation so it may sound horribly inaccurate and inconsistent with my previous advice on precision. However, it's better to underestimate total number of calories you've burned than to overestimate the number and end up not losing the extra fat.

Establishing a Calorie Baseline

Ultimately, whether you use a heart monitor or you use the gym equipment's estimation is not the most important thing. What is most important is that as you follow my transformation program you are establishing a calorie baseline. Establishing that baseline is a key part of getting dialed in.

For example, let's say that your nutrition plan allows you to consume 2300 calories a day. After running 30 minutes on the treadmill, the output displays 450 calories burned. Don't record 450 calories in your calorie counter. Record, as I've suggested a more modest and more accurate two thirds of the machine's output, 300 calories burned.

Record your calories burned from doing cardio exercise this way daily, and your weight, and then log them at the end of each week. Monitor how your body weight changes in relationship to your net daily calorie consumption. Over time, as you record your calories burned and track calories consumed while transforming your body you'll establish a net calorie baseline. Your personal calorie baseline will be your knowledge that as you eat X calories and burn Y calories, you will lose Z amount of weight per week. As you move along towards your fitness objective, you'll see your own weight loss trends on a weekly basis. This is why establishing and knowing your calorie baseline is important. Once you have a good handle on your baseline, you will know at what point you are truly in calorie deficit. You will know exactly how to lose or gain weight by controlling calories in and out. This knowledge will give you the power to tweak your weight and body composition however you chose.

Why am I spending so much time talking about dialing in your calorie baseline? Because it's a key component of not just getting to your initial phase of the 12 week program, but for maintaining and tweaking your weight, your body composition goals and your new healthy lifestyle as you continue into the future. If, as time passes, you feel you want to either speed up or slow down your weight loss, you can begin to tweak one or both of the two variables in the equation (calories burned and calories consumed).

I'll use my own experience as an example. I've been using the same online/app-based calorie counter for a couple of years (MyFitnessPal). I also have a menu of established foods (conveniently stored in the app) that I choose from to create my meal plans. I also know exactly how many calories a particular cardio exercise will burn. Because I have that well-established calorie baseline, I now know how to tweak my weight by making small changes in my net calorie consumption. I can make small changes in the calories I burn and/or consume in order to lose fat or gain weight immediately. As a Men's Physique competitor, this is extremely useful to me. When I'm leaning out for a show, I know exactly what changes to make to my total calorie consumption and cardio training to get ripped. If I need to lose a pound a week in order to get where I need to be, I know exactly how much to turn these two dials. In the off-season I also know how much I can relax my calorie restriction in order to gradually put on more weight, within reason of course. Maintaining the super low body fat level needed for a physique competition is not realistic year round, but nevertheless I still want to look good in the off-season.

Of course, most of you will probably never take your transformation to such an extreme. However, once you reach your goal weight and composition objective, you may want to tweak yourself a bit for an upcoming life event like a wedding or 50th birthday or a beach vacation. Establishing this calorie baseline will help you a great deal in knowing with a good amount of accuracy the number of net calories required in order to reach a weight goal or a certain look that you're after. Establishing your baseline will also help you know exactly where you need to be to maintain and continue to develop your new improved, fit lean body.

You may have noticed something obvious here as far as weight loss is concerned. Since we are eating the same number of calories we burn doing cardio, isn't that equally offsetting? In other words, why do cardio at all? Just eat a little less and you can achieve the same weight loss. Regarding weight loss alone, this is technically true. But keep in mind that weight loss isn't our only goal. Our goal is to Get Fit and Lean.

Getting healthy is another benefit of getting fit, which is a key part of this program. There are long-term health benefits associated with cardio exercise. Regular cardio training builds a strong cardiovascular and respiratory system. There is also an intangible ascetic quality about people who do regular cardio exercise. It's hard to measure or even put a finger on it, but you'll know it when you see it. It's that athletic and healthy look: they are radiant, and they just glow. Follow my program and you'll look this way, too!

Chapter 9

"Don't say you don't have enough time. You have exactly the same number of hours per day that were given to Helen Keller, Pasteur, Michelangelo, Mother Teresa, Leonardo da Vinci, Thomas Jefferson, and Albert Einstein."

- H. Jackson Brown Jr.

Resistance Training

Principles
- **Train to Failure**
- **Muscle Confusion**
- **Technique and Safety**
- **Rest and Recovery**

Your Get Fit, Lean program comprises three critical components: your nutrition plan, your cardio training plan and your resistance training plan. We've covered the first two in depth and now we're going to talk about the third. Admittedly

I've saved the best for last: resistance training. In my opinion, weight training is the most fun part of the program. I remember the first time I walked into a weight training gym as a skinny young teen. A powerful feeling of awe overcame me as I saw guys with developed muscle up close and in person for the first time. I knew then that I wanted to build a physique like theirs, but I didn't have a clue about how or where to begin. Little did I know at the time that I'd spend the next thirty years experimenting on myself. I did eventually learn how to get optimum results, although I made a few mistakes along the way. I had no idea at the time that muscle building and fitness would become a life-long study. Ultimately, I'd learn many secrets on building lean muscle then write a book about how to get it done.

Muscle building is something that I know well. Weight training is my wheelhouse. It's what got me into fitness in the first place and is the part of the fitness lifestyle that I enjoy the most. You want to build some muscle definition that everybody will notice? This chapter will show you how. Now that we've reached the last component of the program, I want to go over some principles related to the time you'll need to spend on the 3 components of the program to better put the resistance training aspect into perspective.

Component 1: It Starts with Nutrition

Yes, I know this chapter is about resistance training, but let's talk about nutrition for a minute. Nutrition is eighty percent of the game and arguably the most important variable in the equation of achieving your fitness goals. If you don't get your nutrition right, everything else hardly matters. You might spend hours a day busting your butt in the gym but you'll never even approach your full potential until you get your nutrition sorted out. My Get Fit, Lean program's three integral components of optimal nutrition, cardiovascular training and resistance training are all important. In terms of the actual time commitment to the three, nutrition will far outweigh the other two. Fueling your machine correctly is an all-the-time thing, it's not a sometimes thing. I mean this literally. Your body is in a constant state of recovery and rebuilding. It's a 24/7 never-ending process. Therefore every meal, every snack and every drink you consume, everything that passes your lips all day every day is important. Planning, preparing, and then actually fueling your body six times a day is time-consuming and requires planning. However, I guarantee you that it'll be worth the effort. Optimal fuel will help your body recover and rebuild after the cardio and resistance training that will transform you in the next 12 weeks.

Component 2: Add in Some Cardio

Your cardio work will be less of a time hog than the time you spend preparing food and eating your meals. Cardio training will require 30 to 60 minutes a day for 4 to 6 days a week. You may want or need to spend up to 7 days a week initially, depending on how much body fat you need to shed. The time you devote to cardio is an important consideration, and the level of intensity at which you perform your cardio training is also an important variable. You want to work hard with focus and intensity, and not spend hours at it. In terms of time spent, nutrition will likely be the most time consuming, followed by cardio training, and last but not least, your resistance training.

Component 3: Resistance Training

Resistance training will surprisingly require the least amount of actual time. This may sound counterintuitive, but when it comes to time spent lifting weights, less is more. Minimal time is required to get optimal results. In my program, you'll only need to do three sets of three different exercises or exercise combinations per muscle per workout. You will isolate and train each muscle just once a week. If you focus, you can accomplish this in just twenty minutes per muscle group - seriously, this is *not* hype from an infomercial. Just 5 minutes of warming up and 15 minutes of intense resistance training is all that you need. Spending more time than is necessary doing resistance training is not helpful. In fact, too much training can be harmful. A big mistake that many people make, some new to resistance training, some long-time gym regulars, is over-training - which is training too much for too long. The key, to be sure, is that resistance training should be done with the highest possible intensity. Once completed, however, adequate rest and recovery are vital for optimum muscle repair and development. Think of it like pruning a shrubbery. You clip it back a little, then when you allow it to recover and regrow. It comes back thicker, fuller, and stronger than it was originally.

As we established earlier in the book, your goal isn't merely to lose weight and tone whatever existing muscle you've got. Your goal is to change your body composition. This means not only losing your excess body fat, but also adding lean, sculpted muscle. Adding lean muscle can mean different things to different people. Building lean muscle may especially mean something very different to men than it does to women. Most guys immediately like the idea of putting on some lean muscle. To the guys worried about putting on "too much muscle" don't worry. You're not going to end up looking like one of those humungous pro bodybuilders on the cover of muscle magazines. In order to put on that kind of unnatural mass, competitive pro bodybuilders hit the pharmacy pretty hard (aka, take steroids, "juice," "sauce," or "gear"). Few men have the natural testosterone levels to grow anywhere near that size, naturally.

Women and Weight Training: The "Too Much Muscle" Myth

For women, the same holds true. Women are often concerned that lifting weights or doing weight training will make them look like small versions of male bodybuilders. Fear not, you are not going to get "too big." My Get Fit, Lean program is as equally suited for women as it is for men. *Women can and should* follow the same plan. There is no secret females-only plan. All of the same principles that apply to men also hold true for women. Developing lean muscle on a woman in reality means improving her feminine shape. Ladies, with very rare exceptions, your potential for adding lean muscle mass (*ie*, growing large bodybuilder-looking muscles) is extremely unlikely. Women simply don't have the naturally occurring testosterone levels required to do so. But that doesn't mean that you don't have the potential to improve your physique with serious resistance training. You most certainly do. The vast majority of women just lack the natural capacity to build freakish muscle mass. My assumption is that most of you will be ok with that.

The Female Figure

Consider for a moment the classic hourglass figure. To most people this is thought of as the ideal female form. Widening the shoulders, developing an athletic V-shaped back, narrowing the waist, and rounding out the glutes all enhance that female form. Achieving definition in the arms and legs will finish out the fit, athletic look that you see on female fitness models who grace the covers of women's fitness and shape magazines. All this can be achieved through proper nutrition, cardio training and resistance training. So there's no need to be afraid to lift weights, if you're concerned about it. Lifting weights will get you fit, and fit is sexy.

In order to illustrate why it's important for all women to do resistance training, consider this. If you were to go to a bodybuilding show, you'd see many different competition categories. Traditional women's bodybuilding (wherein women have built large muscles, typically through steroid use) is declining in popularity. Fewer and fewer women are competing in bodybuilding these days. Instead, they are competing in what's called Women's Physique, which isn't very different really, but it requires a little less muscle than bodybuilding and slightly more stylish posing routines. However, two other competition categories, Women's Figure and Women's Bikini, along with Men's Physique have exploded in popularity in recent years. Why? Because the Women's Figure competitors aren't supposed to be overly muscular, and instead are judged by having well-shaped, athletic-looking bodies. The Women's Bikini competitors aren't supposed to have any overt muscle development but instead are judged on their curves and feminine shape, symmetry, and muscle hardness. Bikini competitors are going for more of the traditional hourglass feminine shape but with firm muscularity. My point in describing these female competitors is this: the Women's Figure competitors, and even the Women's Bikini competitors, will get points taken off for overt muscle development, yet they all are using resistance training to develop their physiques to an athletic and shapely ideal. Weight training improves the female form, period.

Developing lean muscle tissue also helps you burn more calories. Think of your body's muscle tissue as a furnace. Muscle is a running engine that burns calories for fuel. The more lean muscle you build, the more calories your body burns.

The Pump

As noted earlier, of the three Get Fit, Lean program components, weight training is in my opinion the most fun. There are only a few things that feel better than getting your blood flowing into your muscles. Achieving that pump while doing your resistance training feels great both physically and psychologically. When our blood is flowing and our muscles are pumped is when I think we look and feel our best. Arnold Schwarzenegger, in his famous film "Pumping Iron," likened getting a pump to having an orgasm – and who doesn't like *that*? It's also great for our self-esteem and ego. I love it, and soon, when you start to see – and feel – the results, you'll love it too! This chapter contains my complete resistance training philosophies and routines. It's designed to optimize your time while achieving maximum results and will make you look and feel great.

Old School Resistance Training

One day soon when the hardbound 2nd edition of *Get Fit, Lean and Keep Your Day Job* is flying off bookstore shelves worldwide and leading Kindle downloads by a mile, I hope my most critical review reads something like this:

"Although JD's eloquent prose is a real page turner, compelling, and impossible to put down, his muscle development plan sets fitness training back forty years to the 1970's Venice Beach era. JD's resistance training plan is old school. His lean muscle building methods haven't been mainstream, popular, fashionable, or 'in vogue' for decades."

My responses to this scathing literary review will me an emphatic, absolutely true. Heck yes, my plan is most certainly old school!

As far as building lean muscle goes, there is nothing new under the sun. Ask anyone whose livelihood, chosen sport, fitness hobby, or exercise passion depends on building muscle *how* he or she built his or her muscle. They will tell you they developed lean muscle doing intense resistance training, period. Ask the fitness model posing alongside the in-home, all-in-one rubber band gym system you see advertised on late night TV. We've all seen the buffed fitness models pretending for the camera to work out on some cheap gimmick machine. In reality, they built their lean physique doing traditional resistance training exercises in a gym just like the one you probably belong to.

Yes, the resistance-training component of the Get Fit, Lean program is indeed "old school." My resistance training method is based on muscle isolation and intense training to failure. This is basically old school bodybuilding. It's also the optimum weight training method that develops muscle most efficiently. There are those who advocate *always* working multiple body parts simultaneously. Popular catchy terms like "functional movements" are used to describe these workout styles. Yes, strengthening your core while you perform muscle isolation exercises is certainly a benefit. For example, using the TRXÒ Suspension TrainingÒ system does work your core as well as the muscle or muscle group you are targeting. Although most of my weight training exercises are traditional, I also incorporate some type of bodyweight exercise into my workout routine nearly every day. Think of my plan as a mix of old school with a few modern concepts thrown in.

I think that functional movements are great, but my plan doesn't waste your time trying to do them in a weight training gym. Wouldn't you rather do something real? Strap on a pair of downhill skis, hop on a mountain bike, play pick-up basketball, soccer, and football, join a kick boxing gym or practice Brazilian jiu jitsu. There is a whole world of sports that are by definition functional movements. Muscle isolation and resistance training to failure is first and foremost designed to strengthen and build lean muscle. If you participate in other sports or take part in other physical activities, which I recommend that you do, the muscle development and strength gains you make in the gym using my program will help improve your performance in everything else you do. As you develop muscle, becoming stronger and leaner, you'll find you perform better in whatever other sports you participate in. Strength, speed, quickness, and agility will all improve as you develop lean muscle. Muscle isolation and training to failure is simply the optimal path towards building new lean muscle. There's an infinite number of ways to tie it all together through functional movements, but there is just one way of achieving optimum muscle development: muscle isolation and intense training to failure is the optimal muscle building method.

Just Toned or Fit and Lean?

There are countless late-night infomercials selling the latest and greatest workout DVD series. To be fair, some have helped a number of good people lose some weight and get toned. In general, if you move your body more and eat less you will lose weight. Unfortunately you probably won't be building or adding much new muscle, if any at all. I'm not saying these programs aren't good or won't work – but they won't get the results that the Get Fit, Lean program will deliver.

Therefore, I'm asking you trust me and adhere to my complete program. It is tried, tested and proven to work. My grandfather used to say, "If you're going to bother to do something, by god, do it right." Why not optimize your workout time and reach for something higher, bigger, better, bolder? Don't settle for half way there; reach for nothing less than your full potential!

The Big Secret (Shhhhh)!

The secret to getting the most out of your resistance training, the secret to building lean muscle is this. *Train to failure.* That's it! That is the secret. It's eloquent in its simplicity, beautiful and timeless. It worked for Arnold in the 1970's. It worked for the fitness magazine cover model you saw while waiting in line at the grocery store. It worked for me and it will work for you! The vast majority of folks reading this now have no intention of ever entering a men's physique or women's figure competition. I mention how these people train only to illustrate the optimal method. If your sole motivation for getting fit and lean is to look and feel better, then the same principles apply to you as well. Why not optimize your time and achieve the best possible results?

Resistance training can be performed many different ways. You can train with equal intensity using free weights, weight machines or by using your own body weight with suspension straps. You can also train to failure using traditional exercises like pull-ups and push-ups. My program will incorporate all of these resistance training methods into your workout routines. However you train, when it comes to building lean muscle, *training to failure remains most important.* There simply is no substitute for training to failure. The most effective way to build muscle is no different today than it was in 1965 when Joe Gold opened his first gym on Venice Beach, California.

This information that I'm sharing with you now is priceless. It's truly brilliant. The genius is in its simplicity. This is not my brilliance. These are not my original ideas. I humbly stand on the shoulders of giants. Arthur Jones, a pioneer in bodybuilding, first introduced the concept of high intensity training to failure in the 1960s. Mike Mentzer expanded on the idea in the 1970s culminating in his book, "Heavy Duty." Dorian Yates, six-time IFBB Mr. Olympia winner 1992-1997 and one of the most muscular men to ever walk this earth, put the methods into practice. Mr. Yates famously was reported to have weight trained for just fifteen minutes a day. There is simply no better way to stimulate muscle growth than pushing your resistance training to failure. That's it. Pushing your resistance training to failure is not a complicated idea. Anyone can do it, and everyone lifting weights *should* do it.

It's important to understand what training to failure really means in practice. Training to failure literally means continuing an exercise to the point where you can no longer push or pull the weight. Training to failure means going until you cannot lift your own weight unassisted when doing bodyweight exercises. It means that you must continue the resistance training exercise you are doing until the point of complete failure, unable to do another repetition.

Recruiting Different Muscle Fibers

There are multiple possible combinations of different amounts of weights and number of reps you can do when weight training. Using heavy weights with low repetitions recruits a particular type of muscle fiber, while using moderate weights with high repetitions recruits another type of muscle fiber.

People therefore often ask which is best: fewer reps with heavy weights or high reps with less weight. This topic has been an ongoing debate in gyms as long as anyone involved in weight training cares to remember. Conventional wisdom is that one is for power lifters and one is for bodybuilders. Or that one is for strength and one is for endurance.

The truth is this: our muscles are made up of some combination of both Type I (also called "slow twitch") and Type II also called "fast twitch") muscle fibers. Slow twitch muscle fibers are endurance-based and slow to fatigue, whereas fast twitch muscle fibers have greater power but fatigue faster. We are all different. Some of us have more of one type of muscle fiber than the other. This is why some people are more naturally suited to be Olympic sprinters and some people are more suited to be Olympic long distance runners. Most of us will never make an Olympic team in either event. The vast majority of us are genetically predisposed somewhere in the middle.[50] We have more or less about the same number of both slow and fast twitch muscle fibers.

How do you then account for this? How should you train? My recommendation is that you train them both. My plan will alternate week to week between heavy weight with low reps one week, and super-sets using moderate to light weight with high reps on the next week. One week you may be using heavier weights with 8 to 12 reps and the next week you may be using moderate to light weight with 15 to 20 reps or more. Varying your workouts from week to week ties in well with another very important principle of resistance training: muscle confusion. I'll discuss muscle confusion later on. I want to emphasize a few points about training to failure and the importance of intensity first.

Training to failure means always going for that last repetition. It means going for the rep you can't get on your own. These are the reps that count the most and going for those on each set requires high levels of intensity and focus. This perhaps seemingly small detail of going for that last rep makes all the difference in the world. What triggers your body's optimal growth response is training to failure. Attempting that last rep is critical. Training with high intensity is critical.

If you currently go to a gym, you may have noticed the people who've been going to the gym regularly for years. You may even be one of them. They appear to work out consistently, but they look exactly the same as they did a few years ago. Why is that? Because these people are merely going through the motions, their condition is not improving. They are not making any gains because they are just treading water. They DO NOT train to failure and they do not train with intensity. My plan will urge you do this consistently, and if you are one of those people who has been working out for a long time, but are not making progress, we are going to push you past that plateau with the combination of excellent nutrition and intense resistance training.

The Muscle Confusion Principle

You may have heard the term or read about muscle confusion elsewhere. It's a popular phrase related to fitness training. In the simplest terms, muscle confusion means shocking your muscles by constantly changing up the individual exercises and the order in which you perform them. Training with high intensity to failure achieves the maximum adaptive biological response. Continuing weight-training exercises to failure triggers our bodies to adapt and compensate for the bigger load by developing and building up the muscle fibers. Our bodies adapt by rebuilding more developed and stronger muscles. Think of training to failure this way. You are putting loads on your muscles that you're unable to lift on your own. You cannot do the exercises unassisted, and instead you require help in order to finish the rep because you can't move the weight another inch. Doing this forces our bodies to adapt by rebuilding more developed and stronger muscles. If you stop short of training to failure then you're not triggering the adaptive response.

Muscle confusion is the principle of mixing up our resistance training routines to avoid allowing our body to adapt to familiar exercises and lessen our adaptive response. The idea is to shock our muscles by performing exercises that we're not in a habit of doing. This recruits new muscle fibers. If, for example, for every back workout you performed exactly the same exercises, your body would become familiar with these movements and over time the exercises would become less effective. Muscle confusion is achieved by changing the specific exercises you perform for each muscle every time you train that muscle. You're still working the same muscle group, but by changing the exercises you are providing additional shock value which in turns recruits different muscle fibers. This triggers a more effective adaptive response than performing the exact same exercises week after week.

By combining muscle confusion with training to failure, you're not ever allowing your body and muscles to get comfortable. Instead you are always recruiting new muscle fibers and triggering an adaptive response. Falling into a routine is one of the most common mistakes that both newcomers and seasoned professionals alike make. People get comfortable in their routines. It's human nature; we are creatures of habit and so we naturally gravitate towards routine. However, my program ensures that you'll get much better results by continually mixing it up. Additionally, I think it makes weight training much more interesting if you are always changing exercises around so that you never repeat exactly the same routine you performed the previous week. Changing your workout routine in order to continually create muscle confusion will make your weight training more mentally stimulating as well as make your time spent in the gym much more productive.

Steroids, Growth Hormone, and PEDs

In a book about optimal muscle development, I can't very well ignore the elephant in the room: steroids and other performance-enhancing drugs (PEDs). It's common knowledge that most competitive bodybuilders grow to such unnatural size through the use of a plethora of muscle-building drugs. Therefore, I want to be clear here. I am in no way advocating the use of steroids, growth hormones or any other dangerous muscle building drugs. Testosterone derivatives, both natural and synthetic, not only pose potential life-threatening long-term health risk, they can also cause some seriously scary short-term side effects. People who are using these drugs are trading long-term good health for short-term temporary gains. I'll never forget what my dear grandfather used to say, "If you wanna play, you gotta pay." There are no free rides in life. Also, unless you aspire to be a competitive pro bodybuilder or you have a legitimate shot at playing pro football, do you really want to be that incredibly huge anyway?

Anabolic steroids and human growth hormones also disrupt your natural hormone systems causing all sorts of other unintended consequences. Using these drugs is equivalent to playing Russian roulette. I'm making no judgments here. If your goal is massive size and you choose to roll the dice with your health, then that is your own personal decision. Play with PEDs at your own risk; you've been warned.

You Can Make Gains Clean

You don't need steroids, growth hormones, and other PEDs to make gains and get in great shape. In the simplest of terms, what anabolic steroids do is stimulate muscle tissue to recover much faster than would otherwise be possible. This in turn allows the user to workout with more frequency and greater loads, resulting in bigger and stronger muscles than naturally possible. Steroids and other hormones speed growth and recovery time, allowing the user to get much bigger than otherwise possible naturally. Regardless of the fact that they are often steroid users, pro bodybuilders' chosen training methods are in fact proof of the optimal muscle building strategy that I am advocating. Resistance training to failure is the optimal method for building lean muscle mass, even for people training naturally.

So my point here is that you don't need drugs to rebuild your physique and develop lean muscle. You WILL make gains in strength and muscle development by training clean. By training to failure and incorporating muscle confusion, you will trigger your body's natural growth response.

First, we isolate and work each muscle group just once a week, which allows for adequate recovery. Training to failure on a repeated, consistent basis requires an appropriate recovery period. This recovery time also helps you avoid over-training, which I discussed earlier.

Giving One Hundred Percent

One of the reasons I advocate training to failure is that it ensures that you're giving 100% effort on every set. You see, you can't measure any effort less than 100%. When you perform any given resistance exercise but then stop under your own power before actually reaching the point of muscle failure, there is no accurate way to measure the percentage of your maximum effort. Let's use the bench press, a very popular exercise, as an example of what I mean. Most people do some number of reps then stop and on their own are able to re-rack the barbell. Did they give 50% effort, 70% or 90% effort? We don't know. There is no practical way to measure the level of output as a percentage of maximum effort. Training this way will result in *some* level of muscle response. A person could even work out for years this way and after some time make some gains, build a little muscle, and look pretty good. But the reality is this: they could have been optimizing their weight training and achieved much better results by training with high intensity to failure.

Training to failure is the only true way to know that 100% effort was given, because there is nothing more to give. In practice this means doing reps on every set until the point where you can literally no longer move the weight on your own. Given our example of the bench press, if you've done this correctly to failure, that means your spotter, trainer or work out partner has to assist you in re-racking the weight. In the case of body weight exercises, it means that you can no longer support your own body weight. Putting this kind of maximum load on your muscles will generate the maximum adaptive biological response and muscle fiber recruitment. In this context, the maximum load is defined by doing repetitions until you can no longer move the weight or support your body on your own.

An unintended consequence, or perhaps better described as a secondary benefit, of following these training principles is *time efficiency*. Once you've triggered the growth response you are done. There is no need to continue. A typical workout routine in the Get Fit, Lean program consists of performing three different exercises for each muscle group or body part, and doing three sets of each exercise. Perform each set ending in reps to failure. The last rep, the rep you couldn't get on your own, is the one that counts. This is the key to the secret of developing lean muscle: find the point where you reach failure and hit that point on every set.

Training partners, Safety and Correct Form

Let's talk about training safely for a moment. Training to failure with free weights does require a training partner or at the very least a spotter on every set. It's also very important to warm up adequately to avoid straining or injuring your muscles or joints. Third, it's crucial to lift with proper, safe and correct form.

As far as a training partner goes, you don't necessarily have to have a regular partner to have a spotter on every set. A spotter is someone who stands in a position to assist you, for example, with re-racking the bar when you're bench pressing, or to help you get that last rep if you need it. Spend time in any gym, health club, fitness center or weight room and you'll find out quickly that it's a close-knit fraternity. Whether someone is an out-of-shape newbie, rail thin or a freakishly developed bodybuilder, people have respect for anyone who has the dedication and drive to show up every day, and train with intensity. Trust me, people notice this.

Also, in this particular context of spotting, size doesn't matter. Don't feel intimidated about asking someone close by for a spot if you're doing an exercise that requires one. Other people will respect you for asking, especially if you're willing to return the favor if they need one. It's that mutual respect that matters to people, not how they look or how big or muscular they are. Ask a gym regular to give you a spot. Most people are happy to help and they'll respect you for your training intensity, dedication, and work ethic. You'll soon be one of the respected regulars at your facility.

Warming Up

Warming up is critical not only for safety but also to help you get in the zone mentally. Training to failure requires focus, a high level of intensity and a high level of concentration. You're likely going to be training with more intensity than you ever have. In order to maximize your effort and minimize the time you have to spend, your training time should not be wasted talking, discussing sports trivia or swapping stories about your kids. Get your head in the game and focus on the task at hand. What helps both physically and mentally is going through the motions by doing a few good warm up sets. This gets the blood flowing and also burns an imprint of the correct motor movements in your neural pathways. Using light weight and correct form, always do a couple of sets of the exercise you're about to perform. Doing this a few times before the actual "real set" will help you maintain correct form when you begin to struggle as you approach failure. You will know the movement or path you're supposed to stay on. You'll also get blood and endorphins flowing in and around the target muscle group, thus further helping to prevent injury.

Always consider your safety as well as those around you in the gym. Never attempt any lift to failure without the help of a reliable spotter. Also, never sacrifice strict form for another rep. Swinging the weights or using your body's momentum to try to finish a rep is actually counter-productive to the idea of muscle isolation and training to failure. In Chapter 11, Weight Training Exercises, I describe in detail and illustrate the correct form for each exercise.

Rest and Recovery

High-intensity training requires adequate recovery. This takes us back to the most important variable in the entire Get Fit, Lean equation. Without the right nutrition and sufficient rest, your body and muscles won't fully recover. How much is enough rest or recuperation time for your body? If you are truly training to failure on every set, you should only work each muscle group just once a week. The only exception is your core, primarily consisting of your abdominals, obliques and other stabilizer muscles, as they're involved in many movements.

Your core is involved in nearly every exercise to some degree. When performing suspension training, your core is involved to a very large degree. This is one of the benefits to doing workouts or classes that utilize the TRX Suspension Training System (I discuss the TRX Suspension Training System at length next chapter). Even on the exercises that target muscles other than your abs, you are still working your core. When using suspension straps, there are always just two point of contact. Your grip on the handles and your feet of the floor or with some exercise your feet in the stirrups and your hands on the floor, so your core is continuously recruited for stability.

Consider our body mechanics for a moment. We essentially have two major power centers. Our strongest muscle groups are our legs and glutes and our large upper body muscles of the back and chest. Our midsection connects these two power centers, and therefore bears a lot of stress. This is what is commonly referred to as our "core." Unfortunately, many people ignore this connection of the power centers. Even people who work out regularly often neglect their core. For many gym regulars, abdominal muscles are an afterthought. If abs are even worked at all it's often just a couple quick sets of sit-ups or crunches just before heading out the door. This is no way to treat the important muscles that connect your two major power centers. It's no wonder that there are so many people with chronic back problems and lower back injuries. You can never have too strong of a core because that core helps you maintain safe, stable form and balance your power centers.

Training Schedules

Your availability to train will likely depend heavily on your job and personal schedule. It's important to get your cardio in at least 5 or 6 days a week to keep that metabolism humming. Your resistance training schedule however may be on anything from a 3-day split to a 6-day split. The term "split" refers to the number of days you use to split up all your major muscle groups over the course of seven days. It's how you split up your resistance training plan over the course of a week. You can weight train anywhere between 3 and 6 days a week, targeting each muscle just once a week. You will work specific muscle groups or body parts on each training session. My preferred routine is to split of all the body's major muscles into six days, a 6-day split. The split would look something like this, depending on when your "week" starts:

Day 1 (Monday): back

Day 2 (Tuesday): chest

Day 3 (Wednesday): legs

Day 4 (Thursday): shoulders

Day 5 (Friday): arms

Day 6 (Saturday): abs

Day 7 (Sunday): rest and recovery

If your split is less than six days, you'll have to combine different muscles on some days. I'll provide examples of different splits in Chapter 11.

Through trial and error you may find that you prefer grouping the six major muscle groups differently. Try to split your muscles into as many days as your schedule allows. You'll get the most out of each training session the fresher and less fatigued you are. However, I do recommend that you use a 6-day split if possible. Do so and you'll always train each muscle with more energy, as well as keep your workouts short because you're only doing one body part. However, I realize some people may have a schedule that doesn't allow them to get to the gym 6 days a week. That's why I'm providing examples of other splits. Regardless, if you end up doing less than a 6-day split, over time you'll also develop a preference for what muscles you group together on what days. Some people like to do what's called a "push-pull" routine where they work together the muscle groups that push or pull. For example, they might do back and biceps (pulling movements) on the same day then chest and triceps (pushing movements) on another day. Others prefer working opposing body parts, for example chest and back on the same day then working biceps and triceps on another day. However, whatever you decide to do, remember to mix it up to utilize the muscle confusion principle. It's important to never get too comfortable with any one routine. Confusing your muscles is critical.

Whatever split works best for you to start with and however you end up scheduling your resistance training, it is very important to hit each muscle just *ONCE* a week. This is critical to optimal muscle building. A very common mistake of enthusiastic beginners is over training. Once they start seeing results, they think that if a little is good, more is better, and pretty soon they want to work everything twice a week. Don't fall into this trap. Overtraining is counterproductive; as it will slow your recovery, and can even make you regress. So stick with the plan. Hit each muscle just once a week, train with focus and intensity, and kill it. I'm sure you've heard the saying, no pain no gain. You should now learn to feel what exactly that means.

To be clear, pain in this context is good pain. The burn you feel as you get a pump is a result of muscle fatigue caused by training hard. Good pain is the soreness in your muscles the day after a great workout. Bad pain is joint and connective tissue pain. This is pain we don't want and try our best to avoid. We want to feel the lactic acid burn in our muscle tissue. The burn means it's working and fatiguing and breaking down – so it can rebuild stronger and fuller. If truly training to failure, we should expect to feel some muscle soreness the day after a workout. However, pain in your ligaments, joints, tendons or any other connective tissue is bad pain. If you feel any connective tissue or joint pain, stop what you're doing and reassess. It may mean you're using bad form or it may mean you have an injury. Pushing through existing injuries is a bad idea because it can lead to additional or more serious injury that takes you away from training completely.

Summary

Training to failure literally means failure. After you've given 100% there is nothing left to give. On a heavy weight/low rep day you will do three sets each of three different exercises, all to failure. On a light to medium weight/high rep day you'll do three sets each of three different combinations, all to failure. Additionally, incorporate muscle confusion into your work out routines. This will induce the maximum adaptive biological response triggering your body to compensate by developing lean muscle. When you work that muscle again after a week of good rest and great nutrition, you will be fully recovered and ready to hit it once again. Stick with my program and the gains will come.

Chapter 10

"Try not. Do or do not. There is no try."

- Master Yoda

Bodyweight Training

Last chapter we talked quite a bit about resistance training using weights. As I noted previously, there are two types of muscle fibers, fast twitch and slow twitch, and we want to work both types. This chapter deals with bodyweight training, which training using your body weight as your resistance, rather than weights. When performed correctly, bodyweight training including suspension strap exercises can be as heavy and intense as any free weight exercise. I recommend some great high-rep bodyweight exercises as well. High-rep training recruits different muscles fibers than training using heavy weights and low-reps, ensuring a well-rounded and diverse program that, when combined with cardio, will sculpt your body into that fit, lean machine you want.

Training to failure is training to failure. Working out with heavy free weights is not the only way to train to failure when resistance training. You could be a world class power lifter bench pressing 700 pounds for 3 reps. When the last rep is done with assistance from two very large men, one at each end of the barbell, you are absolutely training to failure. Conversely, it could be your first day in the military and the boot camp drill sergeant is screaming down at you. He's making you do push-ups until your muscles are on fire. You give it everything you've got but on the 88th rep your arms give out and you end up face down in the dirt. Like the guy benching 700 pounds, you've also just trained to failure. Whether you're stacking scary amounts of cast iron plates on an Olympic barbell or on the receiving end of Sergeant Hulka's big toe, you are in either case training to failure. In both cases you are also eliciting that elusive adaptive growth response that I've been going on and on about. By putting a greater workload on your body than you are able to do on your own, you will force your body to adapt. You will get stronger and you will develop lean muscle.

There is another, less dramatic and much more advanced way to train to failure using your own bodyweight that I highly recommend you invest in. The TRX Suspension Training System that I've mentioned earlier in this book is a portable suspension strap system that enables you to work every muscle group using nylon straps and your own bodyweight. It provides the potential to do hundreds of exercises, combinations, workout angles and possible positions, allowing you to work any and every muscle in your body. Additionally, because you are not lying on a bench or sitting in a chair, but rather stabilizing the length of your body, you are recruiting your core for every exercise; Suspension Training allows you to focus on specific muscle groups while activating your core simultaneously. Every exercise is all core all the time. The system is lightweight, extremely durable and small enough to fit in your gym bag or a suitcase. All you need is something to anchor the straps to like a pull-up bar, cross beam, the top of a door jam or a sturdy tree. These ingenious straps can allow you to train your body when you're on vacation, a business trip, or as a change up to your routine to keep those muscles confused.

High-Rep Muscle Development

Before going into all the good reasons why you should incorporate bodyweight training into your workout routine, I'd like to address any skepticism some folks may have. This is a pre-emptive response to any nay-sayers. I'm sure there are those who believe and will tell you that the only way to build muscle is to workout with heavy weights and weight machines. There are those who only train with heavy iron plates and believe there is something magic about only using heavy enough weights that they can get just 6 to 10 or maybe at most 12 reps on their own before reaching failure. They will argue that training with lighter weights where you're able to get 15, 20 even 30 or more reps is not effective. Really? I don't buy it, and here's why: consider the following.

There are many real world examples to the contrary so let's point out just a few of the obvious ones. Take a look at the leg muscle development of any professional cyclist, or take a look at the back and shoulder muscles on an olympic swimmer. Many of these athletes have never stepped foot in a weight room yet sport some serious muscle development. How did they build those amazing muscles? They did hundreds, thousands, maybe even millions of reps, and likely did them until they could do no more. Lifting heavy weights is not the only way to develop lean muscle. Whether training using heavy weights with low reps or using lighter weights with high reps, the common denominator is training to failure. The one thing that you absolutely must do is train to failure and there are many ways to go about that. Remember the kid in boot camp forced to do push-ups to failure that wound up face down in the dirt? He or she had the pleasure of doing that every day, sometimes more than once a day throughout boot camp. You can be sure the new recruit also ran quite a bit, was well fed and well rested. GI Joe or Jane then came home 12 weeks later with some pretty good arm, shoulder, back and chest development. Without touching a cast iron weight.

Muscle Confusion Routines

You may think, JD, you spent the entire last chapter preaching the wonders of free weights. Why even bother training with anything other than free weights?

Well, you may love lifting weights, love your gym, and love the atmosphere. You're getting results and weight training is working for you. So why do something else? The most compelling reason of all to incorporate bodyweight training into your Get Fit Lean program is that previously discussed principle of muscle confusion. Critical to optimizing your development is changing things up. The same routine means working the same muscle fibers every week. Instead, changing up the exercise mix will activate those new and different muscle fibers every week.

Laying Out the Program: Alternating Week to Week

For optimal success you're going to train each muscle group once a week. Whether your resistance-training schedule is on a six-, five-, four- or three-day split, you should still only hit each muscle just once a week. Make sure that every week your training routine is different from the previous week. Never repeat the same workout you did the week before. Don't allow your body to ever get comfortable with any given routine. If you are comfortable, it's not working. Week one should be 100% old school, lifting heavy weights to failure. This should be done using heavy enough weights that you can only get 8 to 12 reps on your own then requiring assistance on 1 or 2 additional forced reps. These last reps or sometimes called "forced reps," the reps you cannot get on your own, are as you know by now the ones that count.

Continuing to mix it up, the next week should be your super-set week. Super-setting means stacking two (or more) exercises together and doing them with no rest in between. You will pick 4 exercises for each muscle group and then stack them 2 by 2. You will then perform them doing 3 sets of the first 2 exercises back to back, then 3 sets of the second 2 exercises back to back. Try to incorporate a bodyweight exercise like push-ups, pull-ups or a suspension strap exercise into one of the two exercises as part of your super sets. For each muscle group, stack two exercises together training with light to moderate weights. That means that for the first exercise, use a weight where you're able perform 20 to 30 reps per set before reaching failure. Do the exercises in succession with no rest. Only take enough time required between exercises to safely get into the second exercise position. Choosing a bodyweight exercise is great for the second exercise of a superset. You'll then perform the bodyweight exercise to failure. Training to failure with your own bodyweight is no different than using free weights. You do reps until you can no longer move the weight only in this case the weight is you. You can use the floor for push-ups, a horizontal bar for pull-ups or the TRX Suspension Training System for a variety of bodyweight exercises.

This basic resistance training routine of alternating weeks is pretty simple yet extremely effective. Week over week, alternate between heavy weights to failure and super-setting moderate weights and bodyweight exercises to failure. Your heavy weeks are primarily made up of training with free weights and weight machines. During super-set weeks you'll stack a traditional free weight or weight machine exercise using moderate weight with a second free weight exercise or a body weight exercise. The most versatile bodyweight exercises are done using your suspension training system. Push-ups, pull-ups and dips are also great bodyweight exercises, but suspension straps offer more versatility and work your core at the same time. With TRX you can adjust the level of difficulty simple by repositioning yourself relative to the anchor point of the suspension strap system, thereby changing the angle of the exercise. Exercising any given muscle group you can increase the level of difficulty until you find the angle or position where you reach failure. Depending on the exercise and your own condition you might reach failure anywhere between 10 to 30 reps.

This week-to-week alternating between training with heavy weights to failure and super-setting provides important muscle confusion in and of itself. Following this week-to-week alternating routine is a good start, but it gets better. We can take muscle confusion to an even higher level. The individual exercises that you choose should be different from heavy week to heavy week. The super-set week to super-set week should be different as well. Now we're talking about seriously mixing things up. You'll never fall into a routine and will always keep your body guessing, which will force it to activate slightly different muscle fibers every week.

For example, let's say on your last heavy week back day you did pull-ups, T-bar rows and narrow grip lat pull downs. Two weeks later, on your next heavy week back day, you should do three entirely different exercises. You could do seated cable rows, wide grip lat pull-downs and seated Hammer StrengthÒ (plate loaded machine) lat pulls (see the next chapter for visuals of these exercises if you're not familiar with them). Another example could be on your last super-set week chest day you stacked bench press and push-ups then stacked incline dumbbell presses with TRX suspension system chest press. On your next super-set week chest day you could stack flat bench dumbbell presses with TRX flyes and also stack incline dumbbell presses with push-ups. Additionally, you can change the order of the exercises, further mixing it up.

The point now should be obvious: continually throw your muscles a curve ball. The same routine week to week becomes easy and comfortable. You are certainly not ever going for what is easy and comfortable. Easy and comfortable does not stimulate the adaptive growth response. What you are going for is the opposite of ease and comfort. You want to push yourself out of and beyond your comfort zone. Muscle confusion. You want to activate different muscle fibers every time you train, week in and week out. The secret to getting your muscles to respond is to shock them. You shock them by doing what is uncomfortable and unfamiliar.

The only common denominator or constant in the equation is high-intensity training to failure. Other than that, you want to change it up every week. I've already said much about why merely finishing some arbitrary number of reps on your own without any assistance will do little if anything at all to trigger an adaptive growth response. Additionally, getting comfortable with the same exercises and workout routines will do little to elicit any kind of muscle development. You get the message. Change it up, keep it fresh, and do something different every week. Heavy weights to failure one week and super-setting moderate weights including body weight exercises the next week. The key is to shock your muscles every week, every work out, every set. Muscle confusion, it works.

Longevity and Training Friendly to Your Body

It's been said that youth is wasted on the young. Back when I was in college thirty years ago, we bench pressed three times a week. We hit chest Monday,

Wednesday and Friday. One of those days, usually Monday as we were "fresh", we would "max out". Max out meant see how heavy we could go for one repetition. Both of my shoulders' rotator cuffs have never been the same. We also maxed out on squats using dangerously poor form. As a result, I herniated a disk in my lower back when I was twenty-one years old. I'm trying to save you from making the mistakes I made. My errors have resulted in a host of wisdom that you get to take advantage of. I learned that recovery is important, as is good technique.

It's like in the movie *Groundhog Day*. I seem to have the same conversation with middle-aged guys I meet in the gym nearly every day. It could be shoulder issues, lower back issues, knees, elbows or some other body part. Something wore out or broke after decades of heavy weight training. The body tissue with the greatest ability to rejuvenate and repair its self is our muscle tissue. Muscle tissue gets the greatest amount of oxygen and nutrient rich blood flow. In terms of developing lean muscle, this works well for us as our muscle tissue has great recovery and rebuilding properties. The problem is with all the connective tissue like tendons, ligaments and joints that don't get a lot of blood flow. The connective tissue simply can't keep up and wears out long before the muscle tissue. Years of pushing heavy weights to failure can take its toll on your body.

Flash forward from my college days to just five years ago when I trained for my body transformation contest. Yes, I trained with heavy weights to be sure, but I also alternated week to week with super-setting lighter weights and body weight exercises. I also never isolated and trained the same muscle more than once a week. I learned to train in a manner that would be friendly to my body. As a young man I had over-worked my chest and shoulders and under-worked every other muscle group. Alternating between heavy weights and high-rep super-setting, my once neglected muscles group have caught up. At forty-nine years old, my back, arms and legs look better than they ever did as a young man. Super-setting and bodyweight training do work. They allow you to train friendly to your body and get real results. Super-setting to failure using bodyweight exercises is a great way to develop lean muscle at any age, and it's also a much friendlier on your connective tissue.

Versatility and Convenience

When you can't access a gym, think about those bodyweight exercises that you can do anywhere. Push-ups, pull-ups, sit-ups, lunges, and squats are all great bodyweight exercises. The TRX Suspension Training System offers a great deal of versatility and portability as well. Unfortunately, life isn't perfect, and you won't always be able to make it to the gym when you need or want to. Additionally, some people travel as part of their job. Bring along your suspension straps and get your resistance training done in your hotel room. Bring your TRX along on vacation and never miss a resistance-training day. Throw in some other body-weight exercises and you can still get in your workout.

Here's a real-life example. I've been on my way out the door, headed for the gym and gotten a call from my child's school telling me I had to pick up a sick kid. I brought the little one home, gave him an aspirin and a bowl of chicken noodle soup, and then tucked him into bed for a nap. I then jumped on my stationary bike for 45 minutes of hard cardio (if you don't have a stationary bike, you could go for a jog or do steps at your apartment building. Get the picture?). I then did a killer back workout using my suspension straps and pull-up bar. I didn't miss a beat. It's like the Boy Scouts of America teach their scouts, "be prepared." Have a plan B. Own a set of suspension straps. It's not a bad idea to invest in some home cardio equipment if you can afford it. Or come up with something you can do around the house or close to home to get your cardio and exercises in. Likewise, if you're going on a business trip, if you can, try to book into a hotel that has a decent fitness center. Or find out if it's a good place to run or jog, of if they rent bicycles. With a little forethought, you can be versatile and creative and find ways to exercise conveniently no matter where you are.

Chapter 11

"That which does not kill us makes us stronger."

- Friedrich Nietzsche

Weight Training Exercises

Ok I've been providing you with a lot of background, theory, philosophy, and practical advice. Let's get to the actual resistance exercises you can perform to achieve your goals. Whether you've never done a single pull-up or push-up in your life, or you've been weight training for years, please read this chapter carefully. If you're new to resistance training, my easy-to-follow diagrams will illustrate the start and finish position of each exercise, as well as the correct path of motion. I will also and walk you through the finer points of each exercise. If weight training is old hat to you, there are some pearls of wisdom for you. You'll take away several good tips, improve your form, learn some new exercises and learn to get more out of your weight training.

Let's get right to it. My preferred resistance training routine is a six-day split (see Appendix B for in-depth examples of different splits). A split, as previously discussed, is the number of days you split your weight training routine into over the course of one week. In the case of a six-day split, you'll have one day a week that you don't weight train. If you're following a five-day split then you'll have two days off from weight training per week and so on. Of course you should be doing your cardio as many days a week as you can, and performing your cardio training and your resistance training back to back is the most time efficient combination. One trip to the gym gets both done and a good cardio workout is a great warm up for your resistance training. I also recommend doing cardio on days that you don't weight train. You'll get the benefit of a good calorie burn while allowing your muscles to recover from your weight training. My favorite resistance training routine is built using a six-day split that looks like this:

1. Monday: Back
2. Tuesday: Chest (pecs)
3. Wednesday: Legs and glutes
4. Thursday: Shoulders (delts)
5. Friday: Biceps and triceps (bi's and tri's, or arms)
6. Saturday: Abdominals (abs and core)
7. Sunday: Rest and recovery

If you've got time constraints that prevent you from weight training six days a week then you'll have to combine some of these muscle groups. A five-day split could be the same as above except that you work both shoulders and abdominals on the same day. If you're split is less than six days then try combining larger muscles with smaller muscles to start with.

A four-day split could be the following:

1. Monday: Back and chest
2. Tuesday: Legs and glutes
3. Wednesday: Rest (or cardio)
4. Thursday: Biceps and triceps
5. Friday: Shoulders and abdominals
6. Saturday: Rest (or cardio)
7. Sunday: Rest (or cardio)

A three-day split could look like this:

1. Monday: Back and shoulders
2. Wednesday: Legs, glutes, and abdominals
3. Friday: Chest, biceps and triceps
4. Tuesday, Thursday, Saturday, Sunday: Try to get your cardio in as many days as possible

Also, try different combinations week to week. **Muscle confusion** is important. Always mix it up.

Weight Training Fundamentals

- **Work Through the Complete Range of Motion**

Working each muscle through its complete range of motion optimizes your resistance training exercises. Complete range of motion of any given muscle is defined as its point of full extension through its point of peak contraction. This concept applies to every muscle isolation exercise you do. The diagrams that follow show the start and finish position of each exercise. The start and finish positions are sometimes synonymous with full extension and peak contraction, depending on the exercise. In the case of some exercises the terms are reversed. The exception to working a muscle throughout its complete range of motion would be in the case of some physical limitation like a pre-existing injury.

In a few cases, our body mechanics allow for a range of motion beyond peak contraction. For example, when doing bicep curls, you should limit the movement to the point where your forearm is at a 90-degree angle relative to your upper arm. That point is peak contraction of your bicep. The contraction is lost and the muscle is allowed to rest if you continue the curl beyond 90 degrees. Stop the curl at 90 degrees and you'll then maintain continuous tension, the next topic I discuss, throughout the entire exercise. Curling beyond 90 degrees, which allows the bicep to rest, is a common mistake. The majority of people I see doing curls are not getting the most out of their bicep exercises. Next time you work your arms, try doing all your curls as I described above. You'll have to use a light weight because the exercise will be more difficult, but if you strictly follow the curl form illustrated in this chapter, your biceps *will* develop.

- **Maintain Continuous Tension**

The bicep curl example is a good segue into another weight training fundamental principal: *maintain* **continuous tension** *throughout the entire range of motion.* You should not rest at any point during the movement, and the muscle or muscle group you are isolating should feel *continuous tension* throughout the exercise. This goes hand-in-hand with working the muscle between full extension and peak contraction. In part this is about understanding your body mechanics, and in part this is about mental focus. As you practice these weight training principles, you'll begin to establish a mind-body connection that will allow you to feel the muscle movement. You become more in touch with your body and know when you've hit *the zone* in your training.

A good example of maintaining continuous tension is when doing two of my favorite abdominal exercises. When performing abdominal crunches using the TRX Suspension Training system or when doing hanging leg raises, concentrate on tightening and contracting your abs continuously throughout the entire movement. Don't allow your abs to lose tension and rest at any point during your set. Do this from the start point to the finish point on every rep during each set. By maintaining continuous muscle tension throughout the set, you'll get the most out of the exercise. It's important that you rest between sets, not during. Strictly follow this principle and you will get some serious abdominal development.

Another example of maintaining continuous tension can be described when squatting. At the start or the top of the exercise, when you're basically in a standing position, you should keep your knees slightly bent, and not lock out your knees or stand up completely straight. First, locking out your knees puts tremendous unnecessary pressure on your knee joints. Second, you lose the tension in your leg muscles, which allows them to rest. Do not lock out your knees at any point while doing your set. By keeping your knees slightly bent at the top or beginning point of the squat, you'll not only prevent damaging your knees but you will also maintain continuous tension forcing your muscles to work harder. Do this and your legs will respond.

- **Use Good Form and Maintain Control**

Always ***maintain control*** throughout the entire movement of each exercise. Strict form is critical for optimal muscle development, as well as safety. Let's use the shoulder (deltoid) exercise of dumbbell presses as an example. Start with the dumbbells held at shoulder level, your elbows shoulder width pointing straight out in front of you with your palms facing one another, as if you were going to clap your hands. Then, press the dumbbells up to the point just before locking out your elbows (but not quite, just for the same reason you don't lock out your knees when squatting). As you press the dumbbells you'll rotate your palms from facing each other to facing away from you. Rotating the dumbbells this way is friendly on your complex shoulder joints' rotator cuffs (our interior shoulders are ball and socket joints that allows for a great deal of movement). It's this same feature that makes our shoulder joints among the easiest to injure. Lowering the dumbbells slowly in a controlled manner to the starting point is as important as the press up. This is true of every resistance training exercise. It's as important to maintain control when you lower the weights as when you are pushing the weights. Never drop the weight(s) between reps. Old school weight lifters may refer to slow lowering of the weights as doing "negatives." I think it's simply the correct form for optimizing every resistance exercise. Your cadence should be slow and steady, in time with your breathing. You should also lower the weights at the same speed that you push the weights. Doing so not only ensures safety and control, it also means you are maintaining continuous tension.

Correct form should always trump heavy weights. Overenthusiastic weight lifters or sometimes guys trying too hard to be macho and impress their friends too often care more about lifting the heaviest weights possible than they do about using correct form. This is not only a foolish mistake, but it's suboptimal and can be counterproductive as far as making gains. The best method to make safe steady gains is to perform every exercise correctly all the time, gradually adding more weight. Much like muscle development itself, strength will come in time if you are patient. Sacrificing good form by using weights that are too heavy for you to maintain strict form will put you at risk of injury and limit your development. Poor control affects your quality of movement and the safety and effectiveness of any exercise.[51] Always maintain good, strict form and control. When it comes to weight and form, think of it as quality over quantity.

- **Synchronize Your Breathing Rhythm with the Exercise**

Breathing is as important as any other weight training fundamental. Correct breathing will help you maintain a steady cadence and rhythm when you weight train. It will also help you focus mentally, which will help you maintain control during the exercise. Additionally, breathing correctly will give you more power, which will allow you to lift heavier weight and get more reps. Oxygen-rich blood is carried to you muscles as you train so it's important to fill your lungs to their maximum capacity by taking deep breaths and then exhale completely. Your breathing rhythm should coincide with the tempo of your reps during each set. This applies to every weight training exercise you do for every muscle.

A good example of correct breathing rhythm can be described as it applies to an exercise everybody is familiar with, the bench press.[52] When bench pressing, you should inhale fully as you lower the weight and then exhale as you push the weight. Time your breathing so that your lungs are full when the bar touches your chest. As you push the weight up you should exhale slowly and continuously. Time your exhale so that you empty your lungs just as you reach the finish position where your arms are fully extended. You'll find that the act of exhaling gives you an extra bit of push.

Power lifters and Olympic lifters have mastered the art of their breathing rhythm. They inhale on the recovery and exhale on the actual lift. This breathing technique will help ensure good form and will help you lift more weight. Concentrating on correct breathing is especially important while doing exercises where your torso is slightly bent, such as squatting or bent over rows, because your lungs are getting compressed during the exercise. You've got to concentrate on making an extra effort to inhale fully as you squat. Inhale as you lower the weight and exhale as you push. Inhaling on the recovery and exhaling on the actual lift is the correct breathing form for every resistance training exercise you do.

- **Practice Muscle Confusion**

Yes, muscle confusion has been previous discussed. However, it's worth repeating. The best way to engage new muscle fibers and trigger the adaptive response you're looking for is to avoid repeating the same routine every week. Incorporate **muscle confusion** in your training by alternating between heavy resistance week and super-set week. Also, try your best to avoid performing the exact same exercises and routine week to week.

- **The Right Number of Reps**

Always warm up first using very light weights to get the blood flowing in the muscle(s) you're about to train. On a heavy day, pick three different exercises per muscle. Using a weight that you're able to get 8 to 10 repetitions per set with before reaching failure, do 3 sets of each exercise.

On super-set week, pick two pairs of different exercises for each muscle. For each pair of exercises, find a weight where you fail at 15 to 30 reps (this will require you to try some different weights to find that sweet spot, and that's ok when you're first starting out). The exception may be abdominal exercises where you might not fail until 30 to 50 reps. When using TRX suspension straps, find the set-up (angle) of the exercise where you do as many reps as you can until you reach failure. The angle you put your body in relative to the floor determines the level of difficulty. The number of reps here may vary a great deal. You may do between 10 to 50 reps, depending on the exercise. Whatever the number is, take it to failure. The key with bodyweight exercises is no different than when using free weights or machines. It isn't how many reps you do, but the fact that you do every single set of exercises to failure.

- **Train with Intensity and Focus**

Measuring a person's level of intensity is much like trying to measure a person's level of pain. It's something that only you can perceive for yourself. No one else can feel it for you. I can tell you that you should train with intensity, but it's very difficult to try to explain exactly what that means because it's an intangible notion. Training with intensity for me means channeling 100% of my energy into the exercise at hand. It also means pushing myself to the absolute point of failure. My lactic acid burn and pump are such that I literally cannot do another rep. Do this on every set and you are then leaving no room for doubt that you are training with intensity.

Although resistance training is predominately considered an anaerobic exercise (meaning it's not cardiovascular focused, or not aerobic), it should be done with the highest possible intensity you can muster. Your heart rate won't likely reach the levels it does while cardio training, but you should work up a serious sweat nonetheless. If you're not working up a sweat, then your intensity level is not where it needs to be. This is where that mind-body connection I mentioned earlier can come into play. The mind-body connection involved in weight training is huge. Channeling your focus and your energy to the muscle or muscle group you are working is part of training with intensity. Concentrate on the muscle you're working during each exercise and channel 100% of your energy towards that muscle. I realize that to some people, this may sound like new-age mumbo jumbo, but it's not.

Concentrate, focus and give it everything you've got on every rep of every set. And remember that it's the last rep, the rep you can't get on your own that counts. Therefore, you can't stop short of the last rep. The last rep that you can only get with assistance is the rep that is going to trigger your body's adaptive response. Do this during every workout and your body will adapt. You will develop lean muscle. Crank up your intensity, hit it hard, and you will get results.

Recommended Weight Training Exercises

The following is not a list of every weight training exercise known to man. However, it is comprehensive enough to allow you to hit each muscle with a variety of different movements. If you only do exercises from this book, you will achieve great results. But it's ok to do exercises not listed here – you'll probably pick up additional exercises from other people at the gym, or it's possible you already have a few favorites that I've not included. I encourage you to work them into your routine as well. Continuously mixing up your exercises and adding in new ones is all part of the important principle of muscle confusion, so by no means should you feel like you can only do these exercises. I'm listing them because they happen to be some of my favorites and they also cover all the muscle groups. Additionally, through my own experience I know that they work well for my Get Fit, Lean program. You'll notice that I've grouped them according to the body parts that I have listed in my 6-day split (again, see Appendix B).

Target Muscle(s) and Exercises

- **Back (Latissimus dorsi/Lats) and Trapezoids (Traps) (5)**

Pull-ups (also called chin-ups), seated rows (Hammer Strength makes a great machine for this), seated cable rows, lat pull downs, and for the traps specifically, dumbbell shrugs and Farmer's walk.

- **Chest (Pectorals/Pecs) (4)**

Bench press, dumbbell press, inclined dumbbell press, and inclined cable crossovers.

- **Legs/Gluteus maximus (Glutes) (8)**

Squats, dead lifts, leg press, dumbbell lunges, leg extensions, hamstring curls, cable kickbacks (targets glutes specifically), and calf raises.

- **Shoulders (5)**

Seated dumbbell press, upright barbell rows, front dumbbell raises, side lateral dumbbell raises, and rear deltoid cable pulls.

- **Biceps (4)**

Straight bar curls, seated dumbbell curls, preacher curls (machine or free weights), and seated dumbbell hammer curls.

- **Triceps (4)**

Close grip bench press, EZ curl bar nose busters, triceps cable pushdowns, and dips

- **Abs (4)**

TRX crunches from plank, TRX pike crunches, hanging leg raises, and stability ball sit-ups.

Are There Gender Specific Exercises?

Technically, there are no gender specific weight training exercises. Women are perfectly capable of doing all the same exercises that men do and vice versa. Both woman and men share the same objective of improving body composition. However, there are particular muscle groups that the different sexes are much more interested in improving. There may be certain exercises that one sex may not be particularly interested in doing and understandably so.

A lot of women have no interest in developing their traps so they might skip dumbbell shrugs. On the other hand, a lot of women will want to emphasize working their glutes (butt). Cable kickbacks and dumbbell lunges are a great glute isolation exercise. Some men, although most women will agree mistakenly so, may not care about isolating their glutes and skip doing cable kickbacks altogether. It's personal preference really, so if some women skip doing shrugs and some men skip doing cable kickbacks, that's all right.

Training Around Injuries

One last note concerning injuries is important. Certain exercises may put pre-existing injures at risk of additional damage. If this is the case, then either perform these exercises with light weights or find replacement exercises that target the same muscle (or muscle groups). In the case of some more serious injuries, certain exercise may have to be avoided entirely.

A good example of working around injuries involves my lower back and shoulders. I herniated a disk while squatting heavy using bad form back in college. Additionally, as a consequence of bench pressing three times a week and "maxing out" (lifting as heavy weight as possible for one rep) frequently, during my college years, my rotator cuffs (tendons that stabilize the shoulder) are damaged. As a result of these injuries I no longer squat or bench press heavy. So instead, I do these exercises using light weights and also substitute other exercises in their place. Heavy leg presses and leg extensions are perfect substitutes because they don't stress my lower back. On chest day, I combine several light weight chest exercises and am able to train to failure by doing multiple high rep super sets. Dead lifts are another exercise you may want use light weights or avoid if you've got any kind of lower back injuries. If you've got pre-existing injuries you can work around them in the same fashion and achieve great results

Back and Traps

- **Pull-Ups (Chin Ups)**

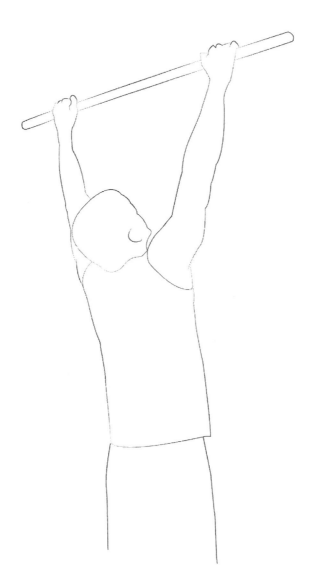

Start by hanging with arms just short of full extension.

Use an overhand grip 6 inches wider than shoulder width.

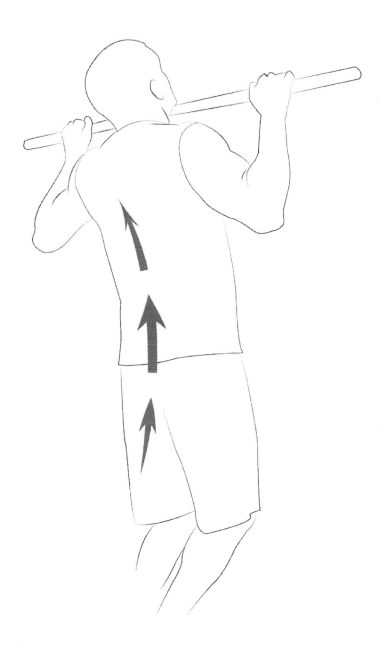

Pull your chin over the bar with control, keeping your legs and feet motionless (it's important to maintain control and not swing your way up using momentum).

Concentrate on your lats, as if you're trying to squeeze a grapefruit between your shoulder blades.

Back and Traps

- **Hammer Strength (Machine) Rows**

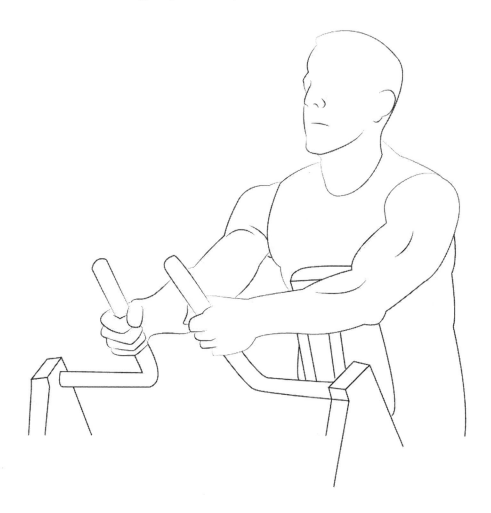

Sit with your chest firmly against the machine's vertical pad.

Grip with arms straight and hands at shoulder level.

While keeping your shoulders square, pull the weight towards your torso while focusing on your lats. You should feel the contraction in your back muscles.

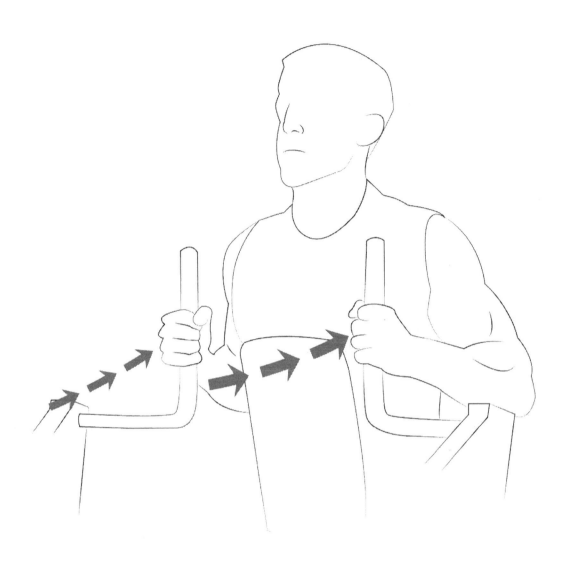

Don't allow your arms to extend completely straight as this is potentially stressful on your elbow and shoulder joints.

Back and Traps

- **Seated Cable Machine Rows**

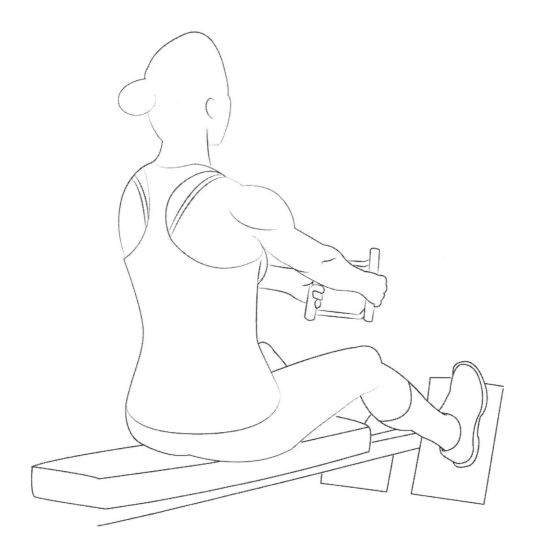

Begin by sitting up straight with your shoulders square, your chest out, and arms extended as you grip the cable handles.

Don't allow your shoulders to roll forward as this puts stress on your shoulder joints.

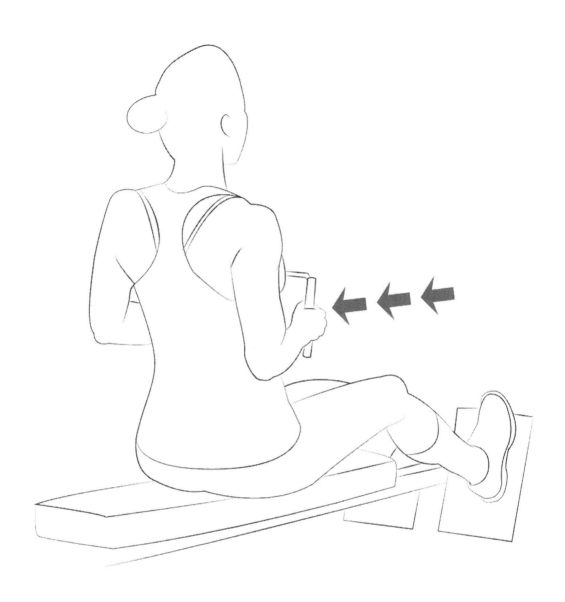

Pull straight towards your body while keeping your shoulders square, and your chest out.

Sit up straight, keeping your lower back arched throughout the exercise.

Back and Traps

- **Lat Pull-downs (Using Cable and Pulley Machine)**

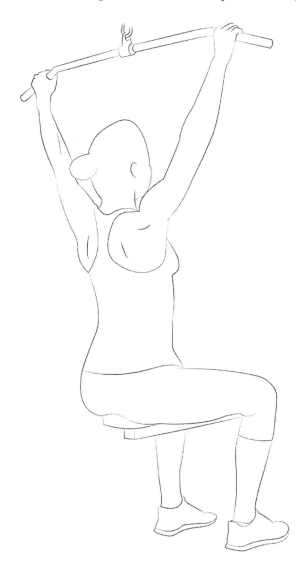

Grip the bar 6 inches wider than shoulder width.

Sit with your thighs secure under pads and feet flat on floor.

Lean your head back and pull the bar straight down to the top of your chest (sternum) and no lower.

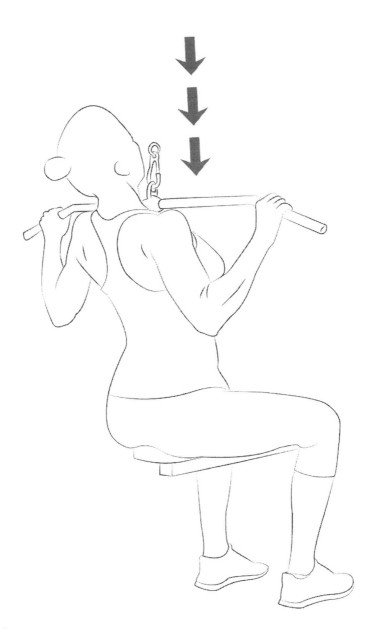

Keep your chest out and lower back arched throughout the movement.

Vary this exercise by changing the bar length and design.

Alternate week-to-week using a wide grip and a narrow grip thereby recruiting different muscle fibers.

Back and Traps

- **Dumbbell Shrugs**

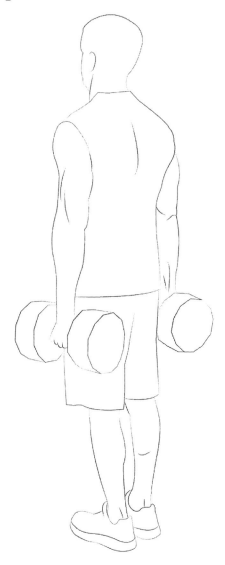

Grip two heavy dumbbells at your sides letting them hang to the point just before your elbows lock out, thereby not allowing rest and maintaining continuous tension.

Lift up with a slight rolling of the shoulders, alternating sets between rolling shoulders front to back and back to front.

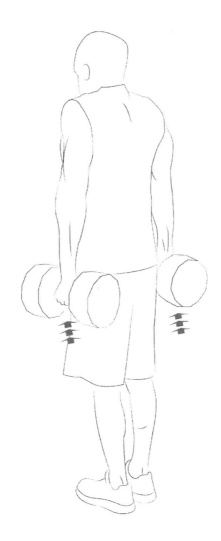

Concentrate on trying to pull your shoulders up as high as possible, as if trying to touch your shoulders to your ears.

Hold your shoulders at the highest point for a brief pause while concentrating on contracting your traps.

Farmers Walk *(not shown, great trap exercise)*

Hold a heavy dumbbell in each hand, as if you were about to do shrugs, and then walk laps around the perimeter of workout area.

Chest (Pectorals/Pecs)

- **Bench Press**

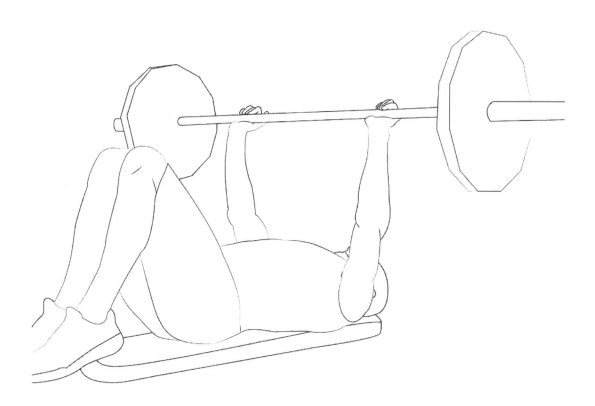

Grip the bar shoulder width with your thumbs either wrapped around the bar or with the bar resting on your palms (more advanced).

Lower the bar keeping your elbows under and same width as your grip while inhaling filling your lungs with air.

Don't flare your elbows out as you lower or push the weight.

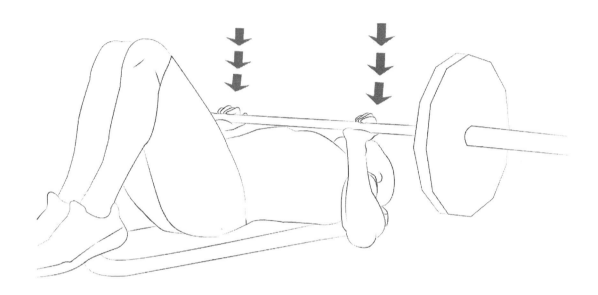

Touch the bar to your chest, pausing a fraction of a second, then push up while exhaling, stopping just before your elbows lock out to maintain continuous tension on your pectoral muscles.

Chest (Pectorals/Pecs)

- **Dumbbell Press**

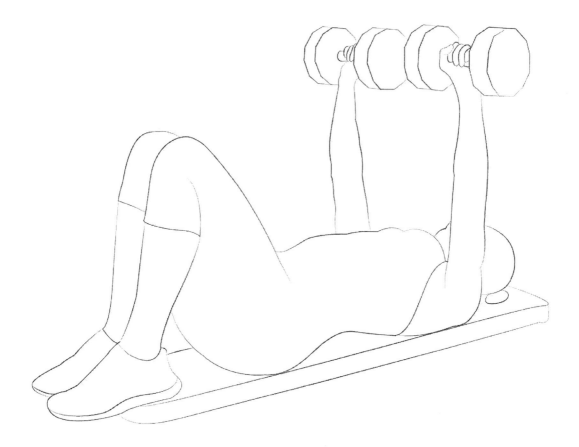

Hold the dumbbells straight up with hands in the pronated position (palms facing away from you) as if you were holding one continuous bar (a barbell).

Keep your elbows tucked in directly under the dumbbells as you lower the weights to avoid flaring your elbows and stressing your shoulders.

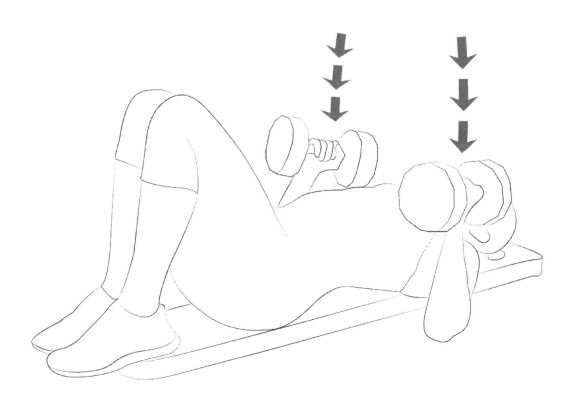

Rotate your hand position towards the supinated position (palms facing each other) as you lower the weight.

Lower the weights to the point that they are no lower than your chest, pause a microsecond and push weights back up.

Lowering the dumbbells lower than your chest is potentially stressful on your shoulder joints.

Chest (Pectorals/Pecs)

- **Inclined Dumbbell Press**

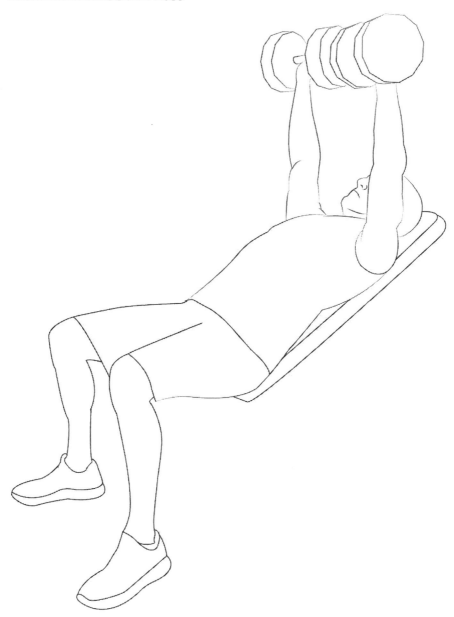

Use the same mechanics as flat bench dumbbell press in previous exercise.

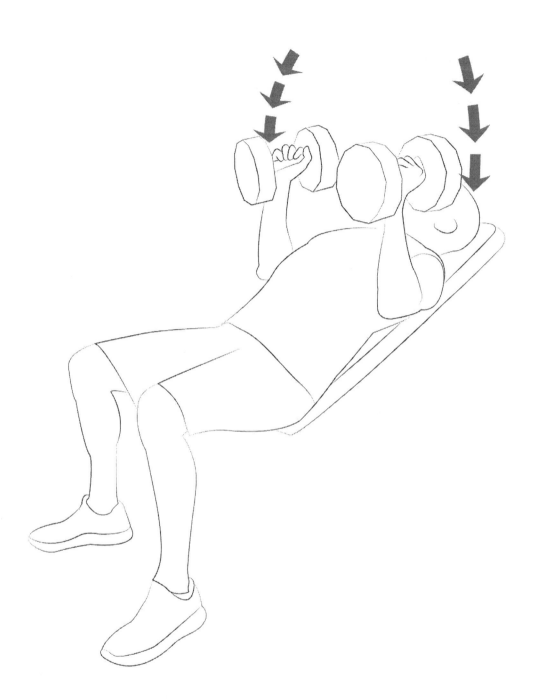

Set the angle of the bench to 30 degrees, the optimal angle for concentrating on the midpoint of your pectoral muscle.

Chest (Pectorals/Pecs)

- **Inclined Cable Crossovers**

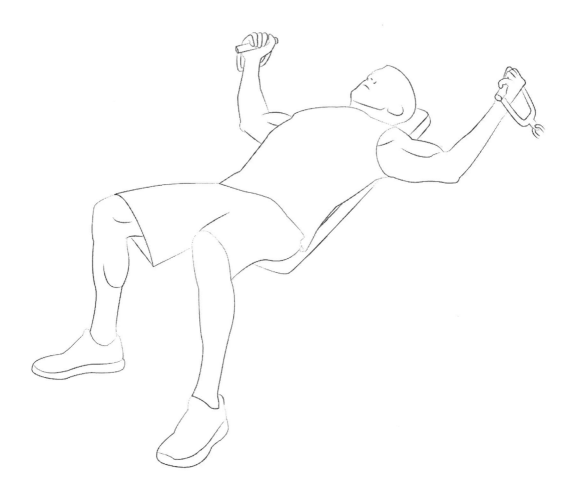

Position an inclined bench at and angle of 30 degrees equidistant between two cable and pulley machines.

Begin with hands wide and elbows locked at a slight bend.

Alternate pulling the cables together and slightly cross your hands, concentrating on squeezing your pecs together.

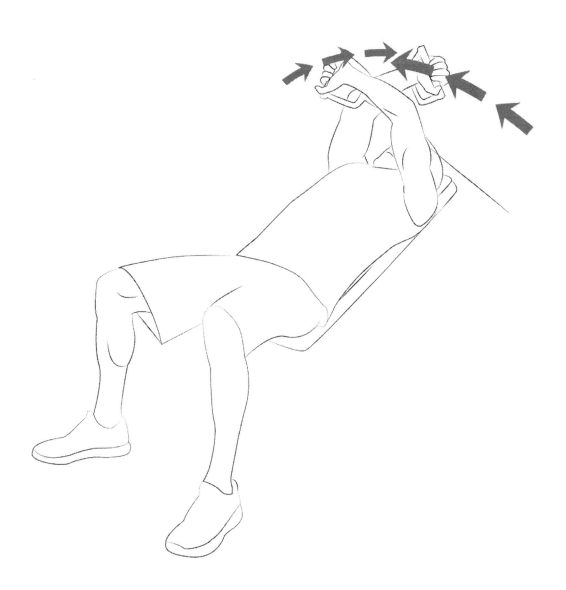

Alternate left hand crossing over right and right over left.

Hold your hands high throughout the motion, making a big smooth arc motion pointing out and away from your upper chest.

Legs/Gluteus Maximus (Glutes)

- **Squats**

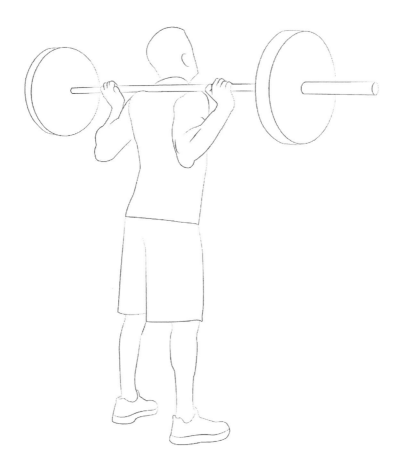

With the barbell across your upper back and shoulders, your weight should be evenly distributed across the length of your feet.

Tip: *lead with your butt* as you squat down as if you were aiming your backside at a short stool (or sitting on the toilet).

Keep your lower back tight and chest out throughout the motion.

Imagining you are trying to hold a melon between your shoulder blades will ensure that you keep your chest out.

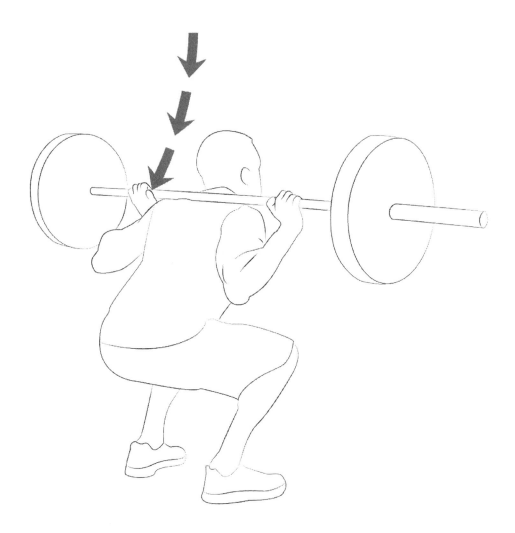

Tip: as you bend your torso your lungs are compressed, so you must concentrate on inhaling as you lower the weight.

Inhale, concentrating on filling your lungs with air as you squat down, then exhale as you stand up.

Your quadriceps should be parallel to the floor at the lowest position of the squat.

Do not lock out your knees at the top, keep them slightly bent to maintain continuous pressure on your leg muscles.

Legs/Gluteus Maximus (Glutes)

- **Deadlifts**

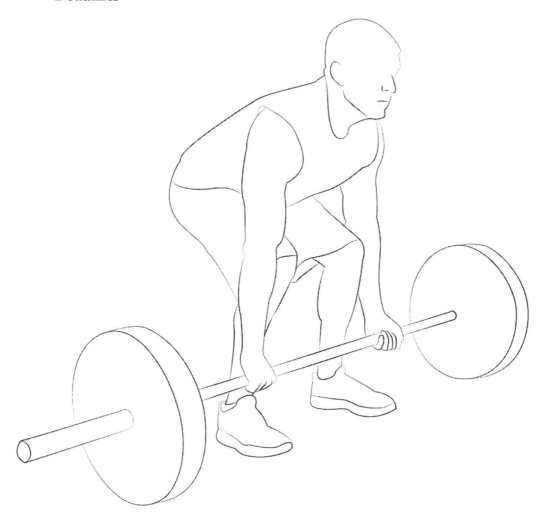

Begin with your feet at shoulder width and grip the bar just wider than shoulder width.

Inhale, filling your lungs with air before you lift, and exhale as you stand up.

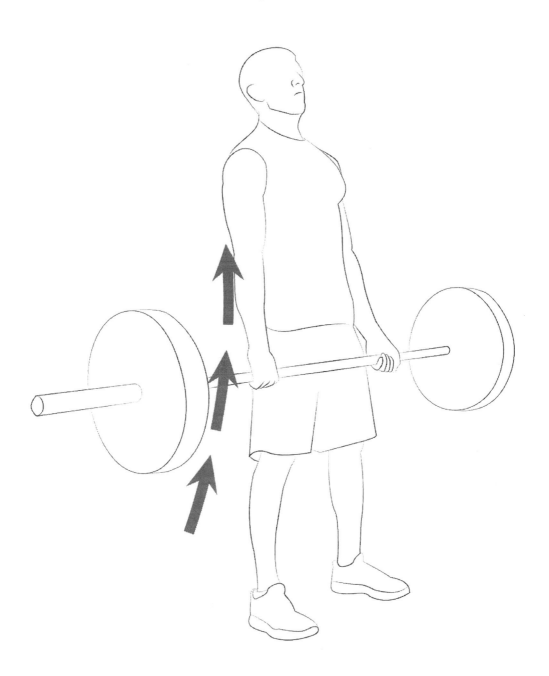

Keep your lower back tight, chest out and head up throughout the lift.

Pause at the top of the exercise, then lower the weight back to the floor with control.

Legs/Gluteus Maximus (Glutes)

- **Leg Press**

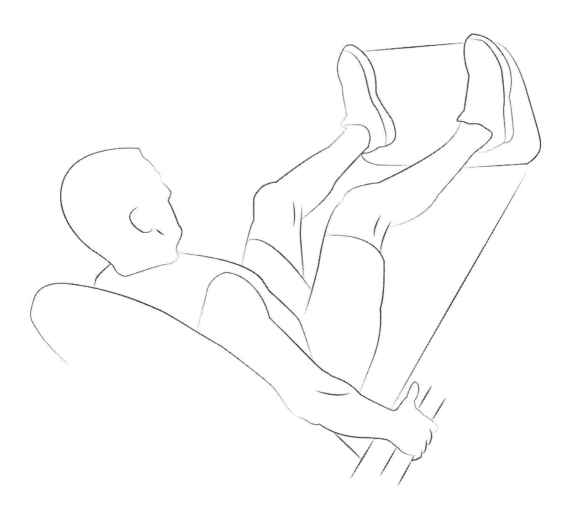

Begin with feet wide and high on upper corners of platform.

Lower the weight allowing your knees to bend back to the point where your quadriceps are parallel to the platform you're pushing.

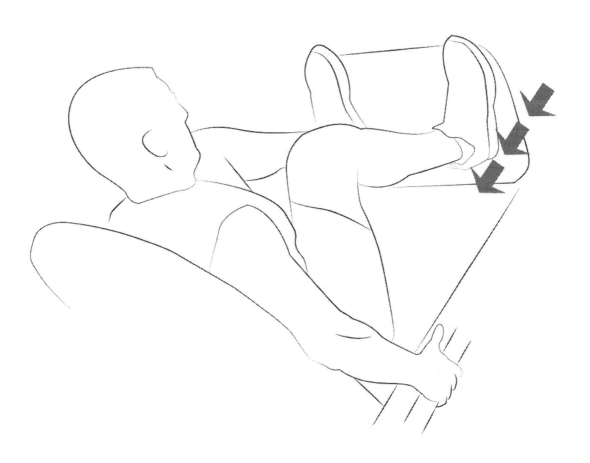

Breathe as you would while squatting, inhale as you lower the weight and exhale as you push.

Push the weight up with the weight evenly distributed across your feet.

Legs/Gluteus Maximus (Glutes)

- **Dumbbell Lunges**

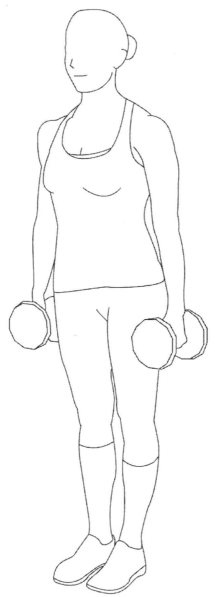

Begin by taking a normal stride length forward.

Keep your back straight, chest out and look straight ahead as the toes of your back foot grip the floor.

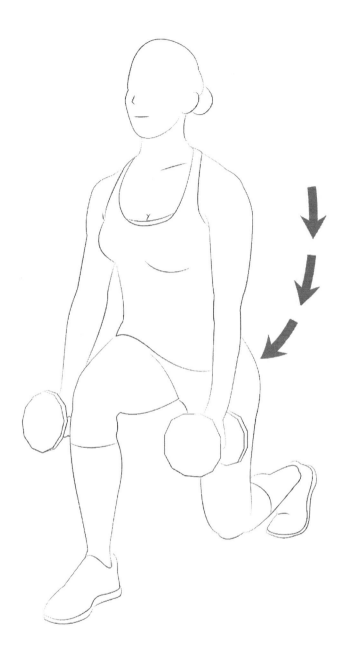

Bend your front leg to the point where your quad is parallel, then stand back up and return your leg back to the starting point.

Switch legs and repeat, alternating legs on each rep.

Legs/Gluteus Maximus (Glutes)

- **Leg Extensions**

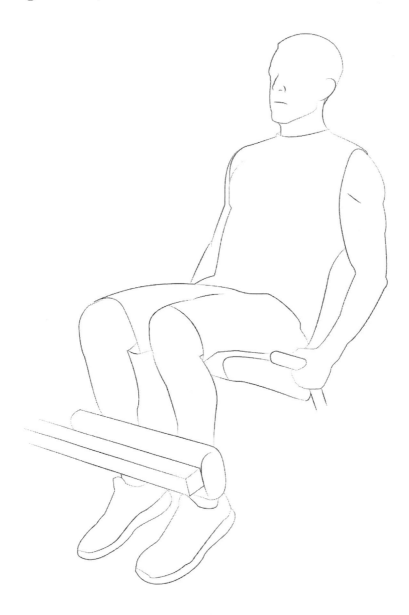

Begin sitting with legs bent at a ninety-degree angle.

Hold yourself down securely in the seat as you lift.

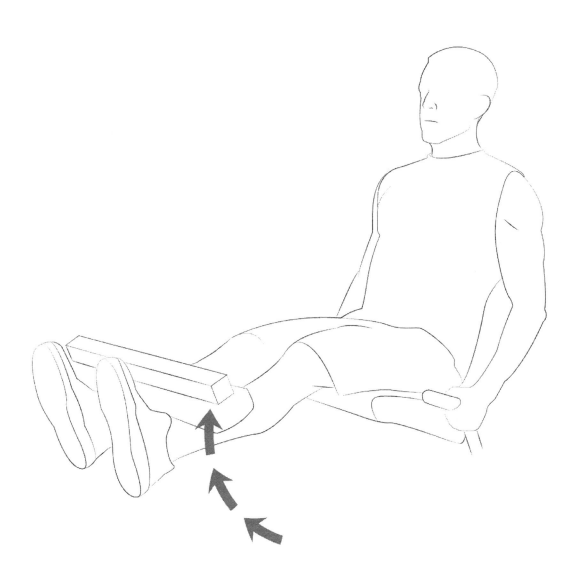

Pause briefly at peak contraction where your legs are fully extended.

Legs/Gluteus Maximus (Glutes)

- **Hamstring Curls**

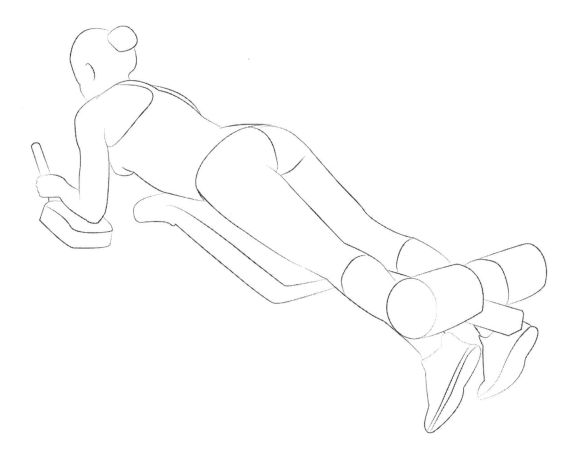

Begin with legs fully extended.

Curl the weight as far as possible while pausing at peak contraction of your hamstrings.

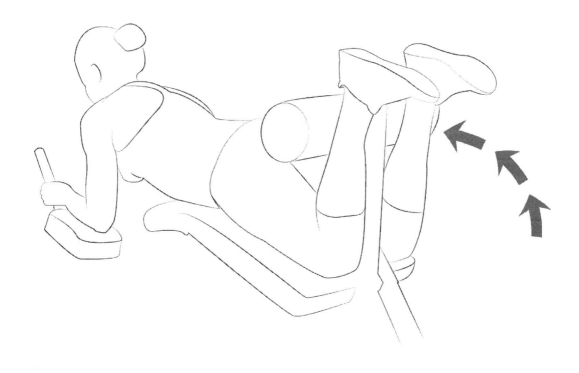

Inhale as you lower the weight and exhale as you perform the curl.

Lower the weight back to the starting position slowly with control.

Legs/Gluteus Maximus (Glutes)

- **Cable Kickbacks**

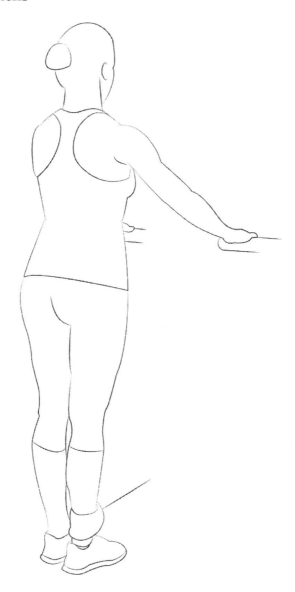

You'll first need an ankle cuff that cable equipment clips into (most gyms have these; if not they are inexpensive online).

Stand up straight with your feet together holding the machine for balance.

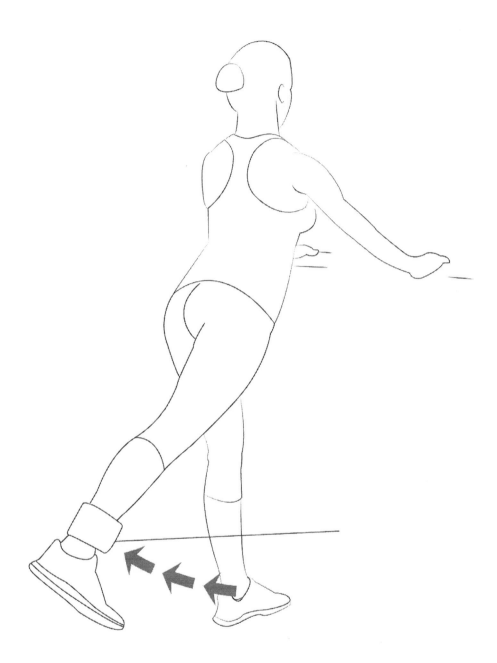

Kick your heel straight back while keeping your leg straight.

Concentrate on contracting your glute at the top of the motion.

Legs/Gluteus Maximus (Glutes)

- **Calf Raises (Calf Machine Raises)**

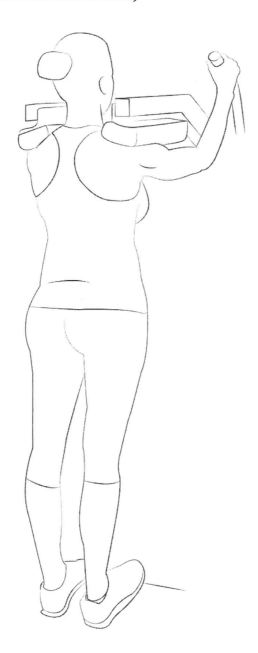

Begin your toes on the provided block with your heels as low as possible (full calf extension).

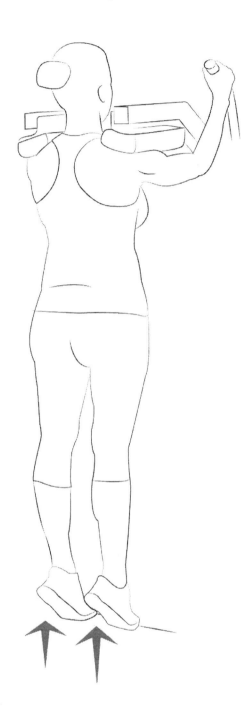

End with your heels raised as much as possible (peak contraction) holding this position for a brief pause.

Shoulders

- **Seated Dumbbell Press**

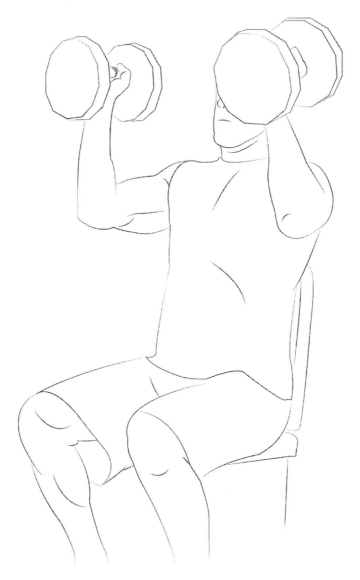

Begin with the dumbbells at ear level, elbows tucked in and your palms facing each other.

Rotate the dumbbells as you push them up so that your hands are in the pronated position (facing out away from you) at the top of the exercise.

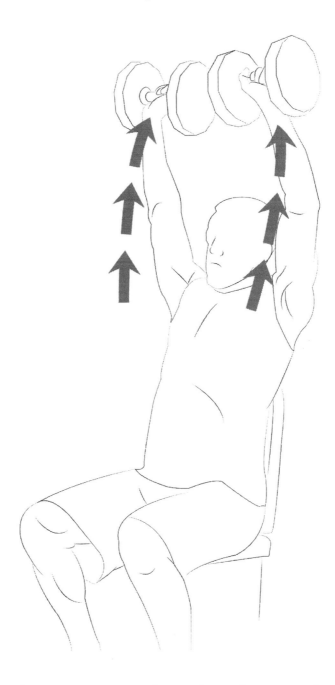

Rotate the weights in reverse as you lower them, then rotate them as described above as you raise them again.

This natural movement is friendly on your complex shoulder ball joint causing the least amount of stress on the connective tissue.

Shoulders

- **Upright Barbell Rows**

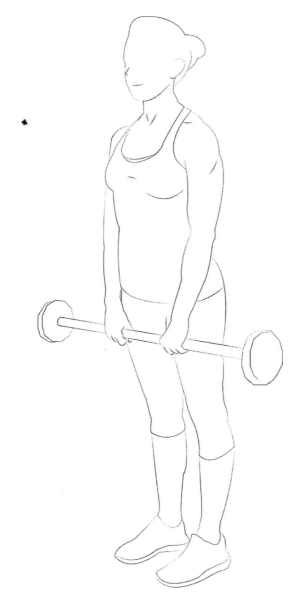

Start with your arms down and the bar against your upper legs/groin area.

Grip the bar with your hands at chest width.

Lift the bar straight up to just under your chin.

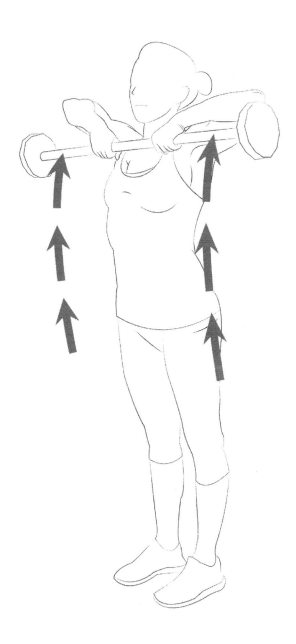

Pause at top of the exercise concentrating on traps and shoulders.

Maintain continuous tension by *not* resting the bar against your legs between reps (hold it slightly away from your body).

Shoulders

- **Front Dumbbell Raises**

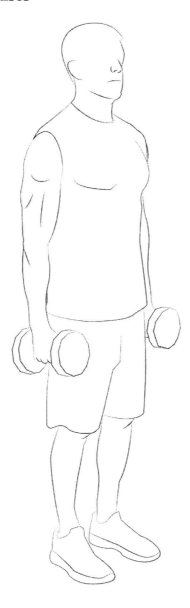

Begin holding the dumbbells down at your upper legs, with the back of your hand facing away from you.

Keeping your arm straight and elbows locked, alternate raising the dumbbells to shoulder height.

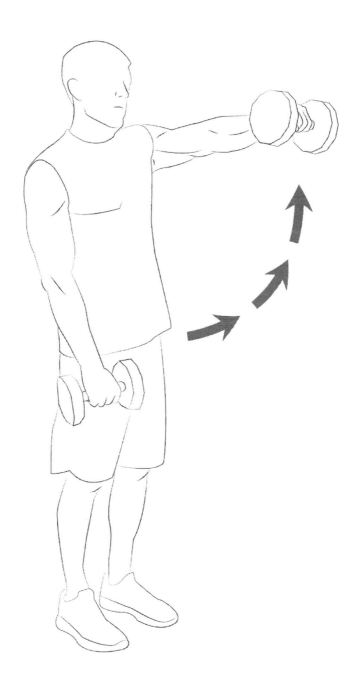

Pause at the top of the movement, concentrating on front deltoids.

Maintain continuous tension by *not* resting the dumbbells on your legs between reps (keep them slightly away from your body).

Shoulders

- **Side Lateral Dumbbell Raises**

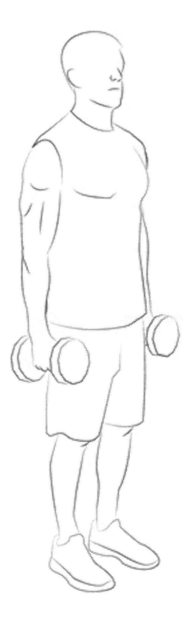

Begin holding the dumbbells against the side of your legs with the back of your hands facing to the sides and away from you.

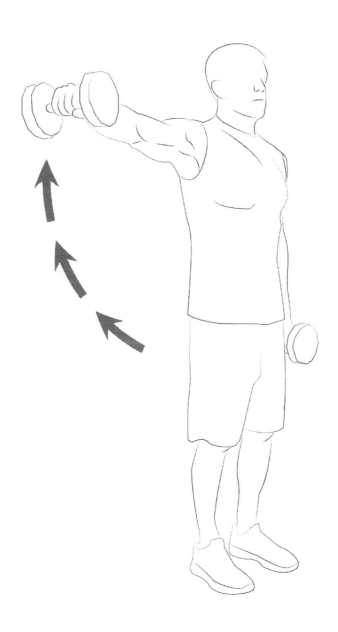

Keeping your arms straight and elbow locked, alternate raising the dumbbells to shoulder height.

Maintain continuous tension by not resting dumbbells on legs between reps.

Shoulders

- **Rear Deltoid Cable Pulls**

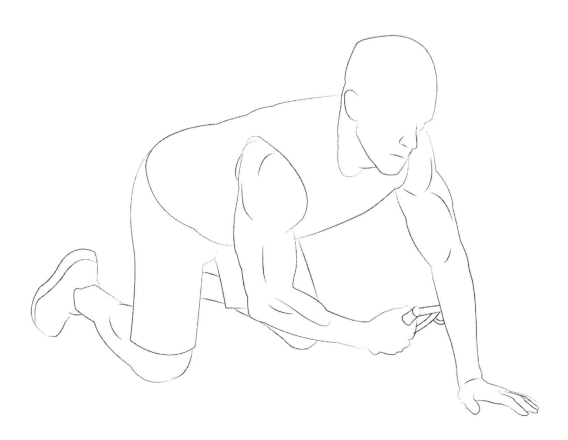

Begin on all fours with your shoulders square and aligned perpendicularly to cable machine pulley.

Grip the cable handle underneath and on the opposite side of your body.

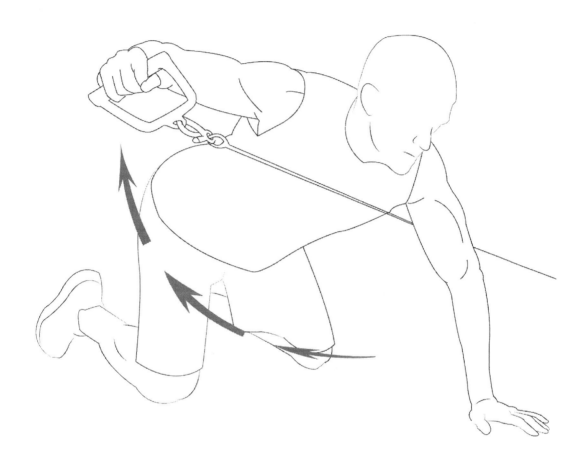

While keeping your elbow slightly bent and locked, pull cable in an upward arc, concentrating on your rear deltoids as if you're trying to crack a walnut between your rear deltoid and your shoulder blade.

In your mind's eye don't think of the movement as pulling but rather as pushing the back of your hand against a force.

Biceps

- **Straight Bar Curls**

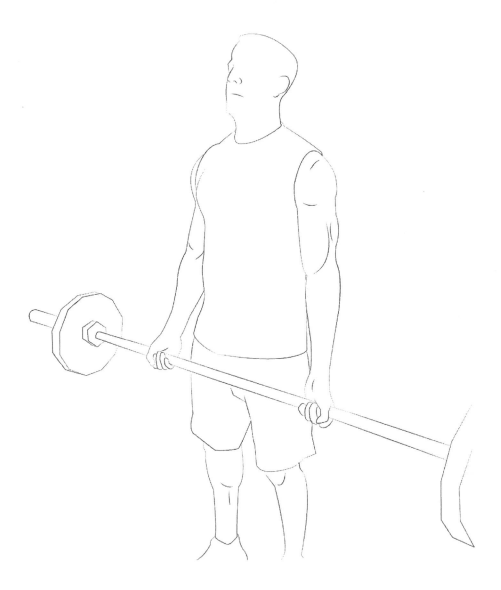

Begin by gripping the barbell shoulder width with arms fully extended, palms facing away from you.

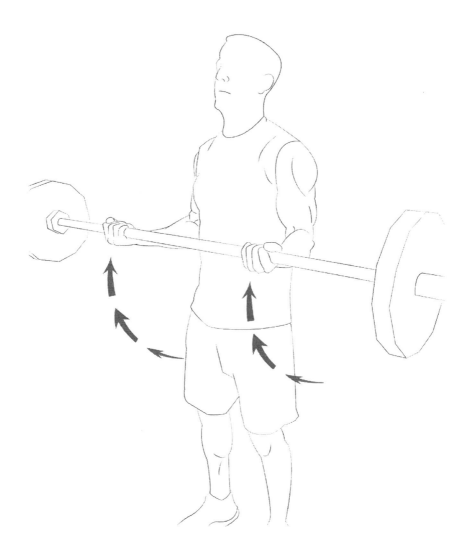

While keeping your entire body motionless, curl the bar stopping and pausing briefly at 90 degrees.

Although your arms can bend far more than 90 degrees, don't go beyond this point (this is my secret bicep development tip).

90 degrees is peak contraction of the bicep, anything more and continuous tension is lost, allowing the muscle to rest.

Follow this form strictly and your biceps will develop.

Biceps

- **Seated Dumbbell Curls**

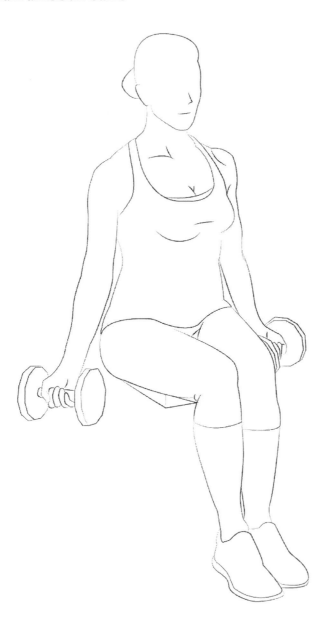

Begin holding the dumbbells allowing them to hang at your sides.

Before beginning to curl, turn your hand and twist the dumbbell until your palm faces sideways away from your body.

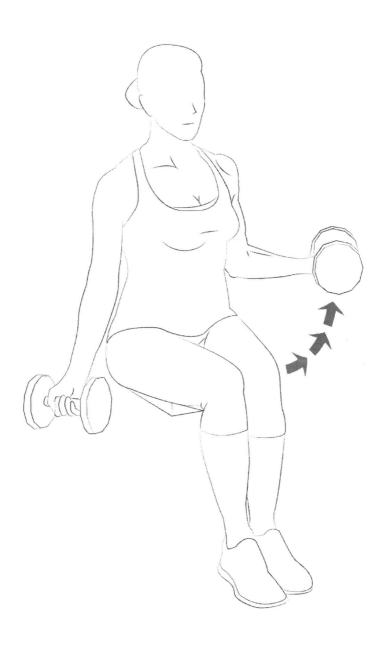

Only after turning your hand you then curl the weight, stopping at peak contraction (a 90 degree bend in your arm).

Lower the weight slowly. Allow your hand to roll back to the start position only after your arm is hanging straight down and fully extended.

Biceps

- **Preacher Curls (Machine or EZ Curl Bar)**

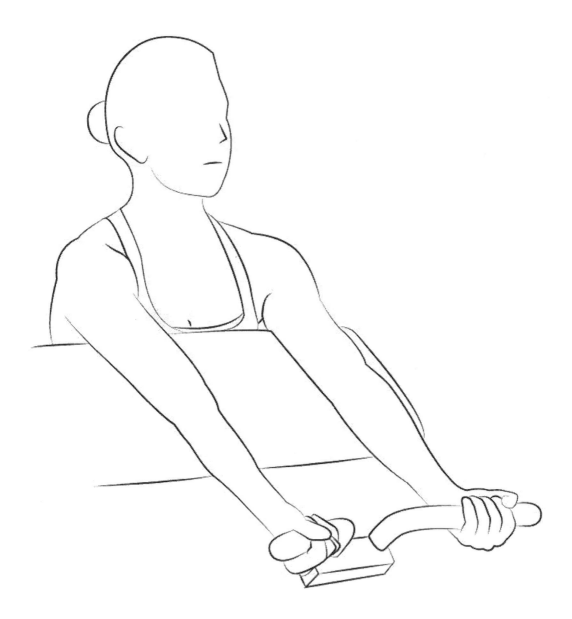

Begin with the back of your upper arms laying flat against the machine's arm pad.

Keep your body stable and motionless, and your upper arms pressed against the pad, as the only movement should be from the elbow down.

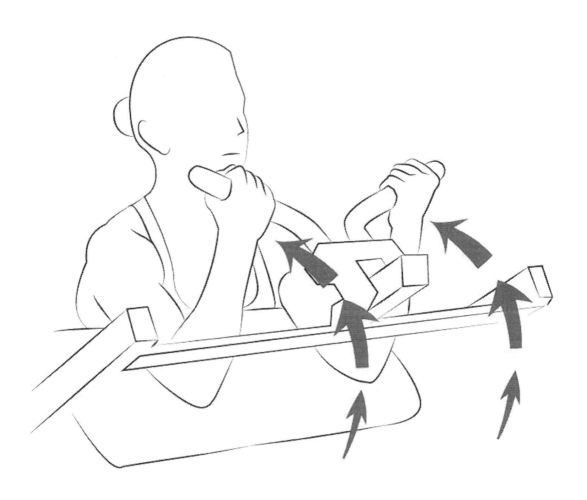

Grip the bar shoulder width and curl, stopping at a 90-degree bend in your arm.

Lower the bar with control to the start position of full extension.

If your gym doesn't have a machine version of this, you can do it on a preacher bench with a curl bar or straight bar.

Biceps

- **Seated Dumbbell Hammer Curls**

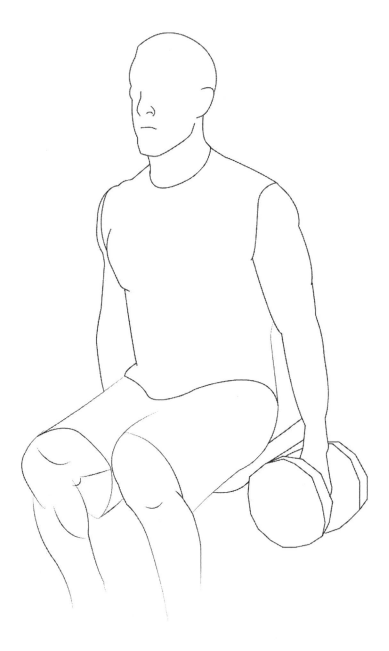

Begin with your arms fully extended, holding the dumbbells with the back of your hands facing to the side away from you.

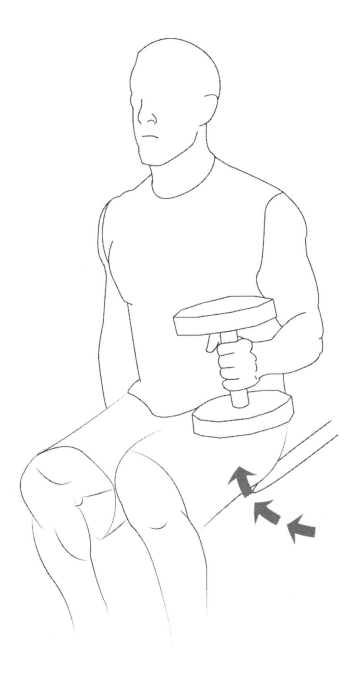

Curl the dumbbells to a 90-degree bend in your arm, keeping your hands in the same position and pausing at peak contraction.

Lower the weights with control to the full extension position.

Triceps

- **Close Grip Bench Press**

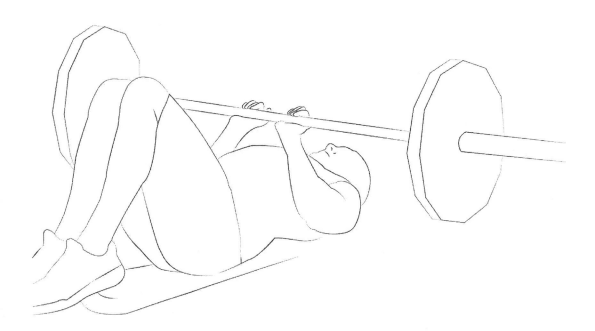

Grip the barbell where your hands are close enough that your thumbs are touching.

Keep your elbows in a shoulder-width vertical plane throughout the movement as opposed to letting them flare out to the side.

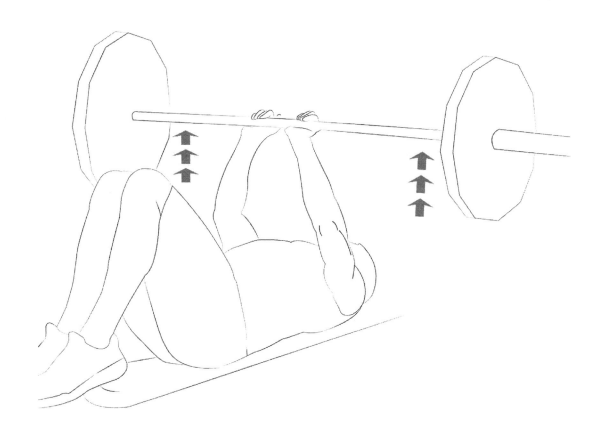

The range of motion should be such that you stop just before locking out your arms to full extension at the top, and just before the bar touches your chest at the bottom of the exercise.

This maintains continuous tension throughout the exercise.

Inhale as you lower the bar and exhale as you push.

Triceps

- **EZ Bar Nose Busters**

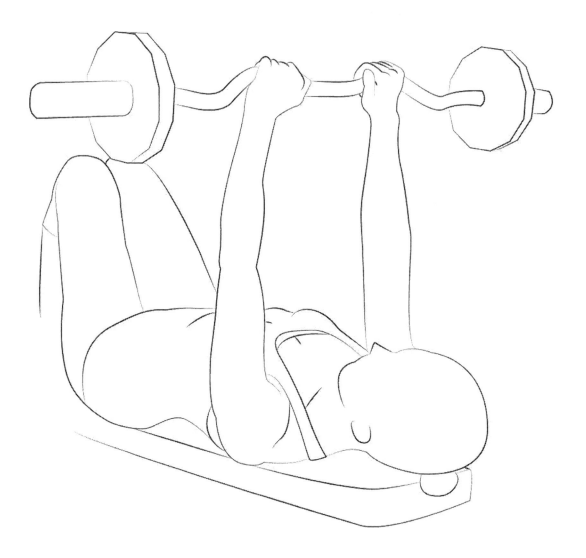

Your grip should be about the width of your pecs, palms facing away from you.

Your upper arms from your elbows to your shoulders should remain perpendicular to the floor and motionless throughout the movement as you lower the bar to your nose and then extend back up,

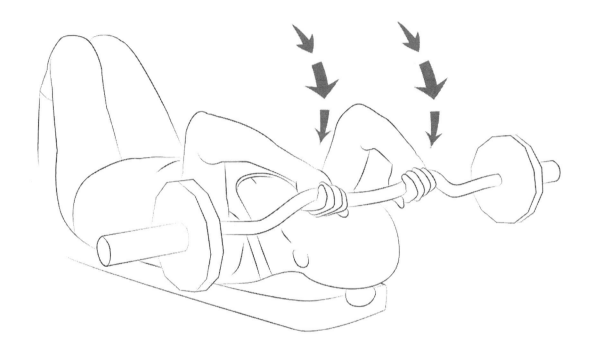

Maximum range of motion is achieved by bending your wrist correctly throughout the movement.

When your arms are straight up, your wrist should be bent backwards and at the lowest point of the exercise your wrist should be bent forward.

Triceps

- **Triceps Cable Pushdowns**

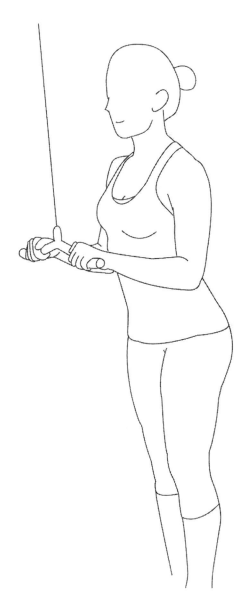

Begin with your elbows bent at a 90-degree angle and your wrist bent forward and down.

As you push down keep your elbows tight against your sides while bending your wrist backwards as your extend your arms straight down.

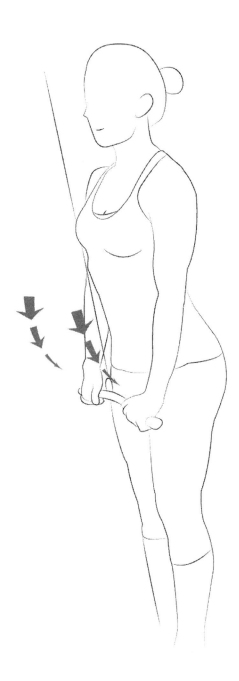

Peak triceps contraction is arms straight and wrist bent backwards.

Triceps

- **Dips**

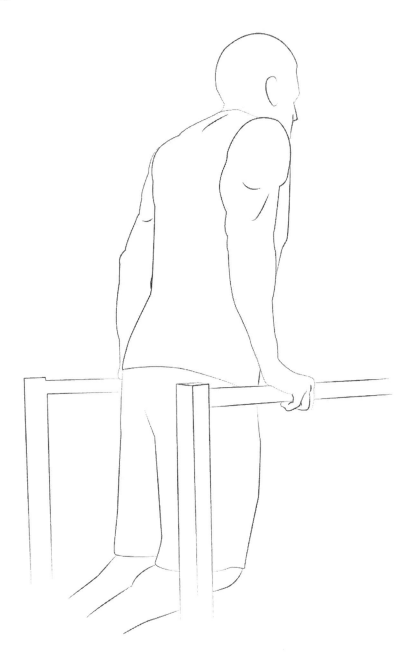

Start with a comfortable grip and good posture. Hold your shoulders slightly back and keep your chest out throughout the exercise.

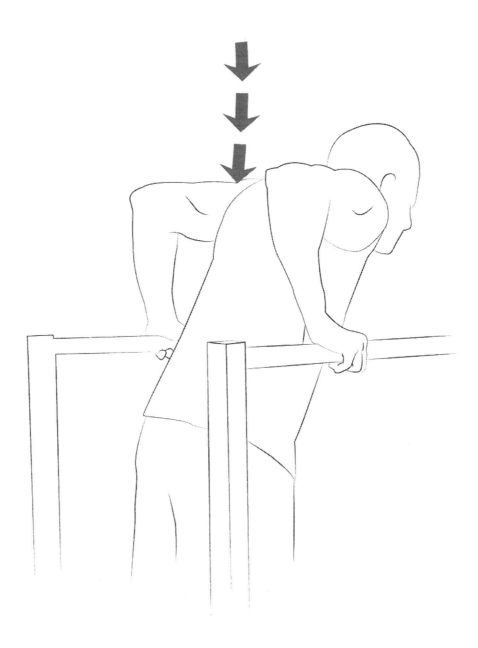

As you lower yourself keep your elbows shoulder width and directly behind you, not flared out to the sides.

Lower yourself until the back of your arm is parallel to the floor.

Abs

- **TRX Crunches from Plank**

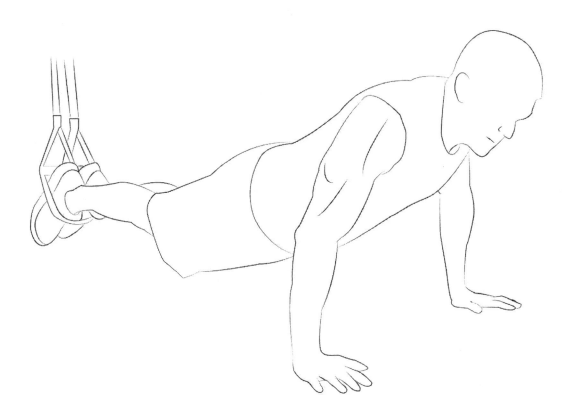

Begin with feet in the stirrups, in pushup ready position, facing the floor and with your body in a straight line.

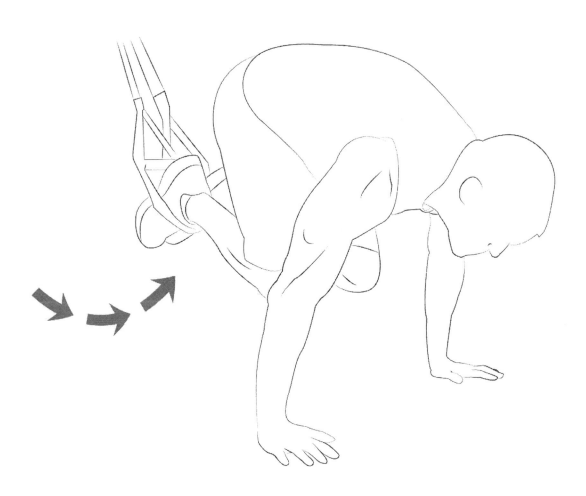

Brings your knees forward together as if you're trying to touch your knees to your chest.

Return slowly to the start position while focusing and maintaining continuous tension on your abs.

Abs

- **TRX Pike Crunches**

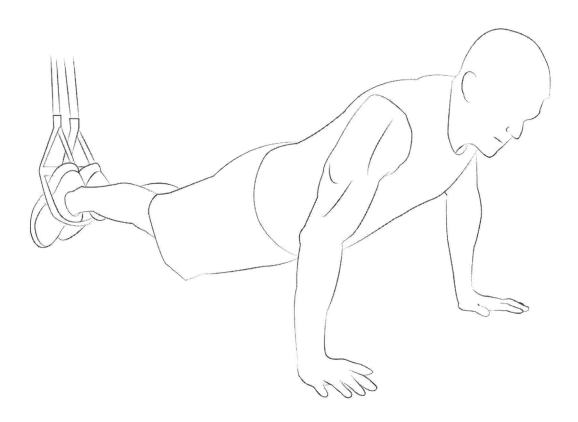

Begin with your feet in the stirrups, in pushup ready position, facing the floor and with your body in a straight line.

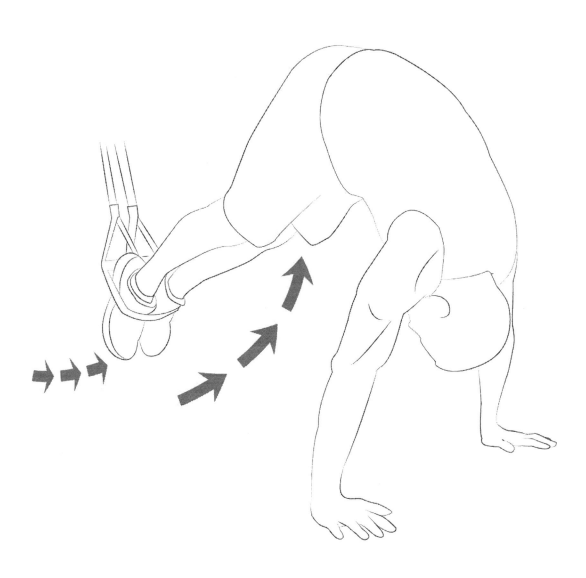

Without bending your knees, bring your feet forwards as far as possible, pointing your glutes straight up as high as possible.

Pause at the top of the exercise for peak contraction, then lower slowly and maintain focus and continuous tension throughout the exercise. Repeat to failure.

Abs

- **Hanging Leg Raises**

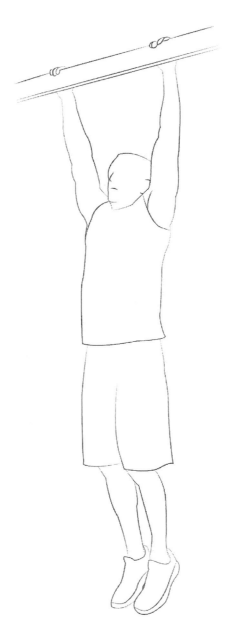

Suspend yourself from a pull-up bar either using your own grip or a pair of hanging ab straps.

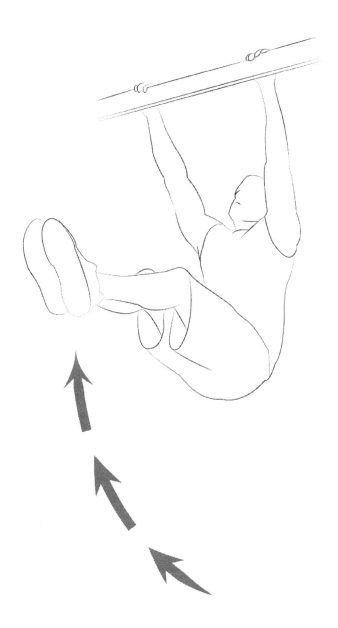

Begin by hanging straight down, then lift your feet straight out as high as you can with a slight bend in your knees.

Only bend at the waist, try not to swing your body, and maintain continuous focus and tension on your abs.

Abs

- **Stability Ball Sit-Up/Crunch**

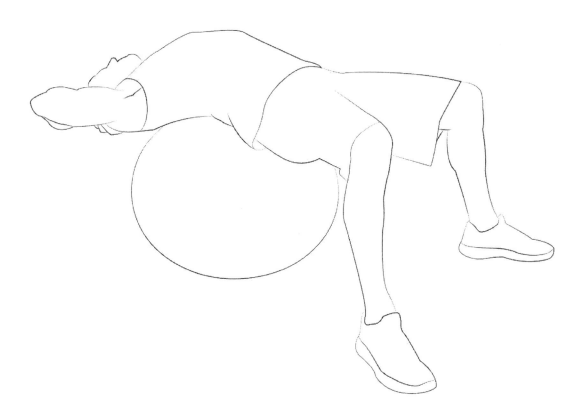

Balance yourself on a stability ball with your weight centered on your lower back, against the ball.

Begin with yourself bent slightly backwards with your hands beside your head and your head lower than your midsection.

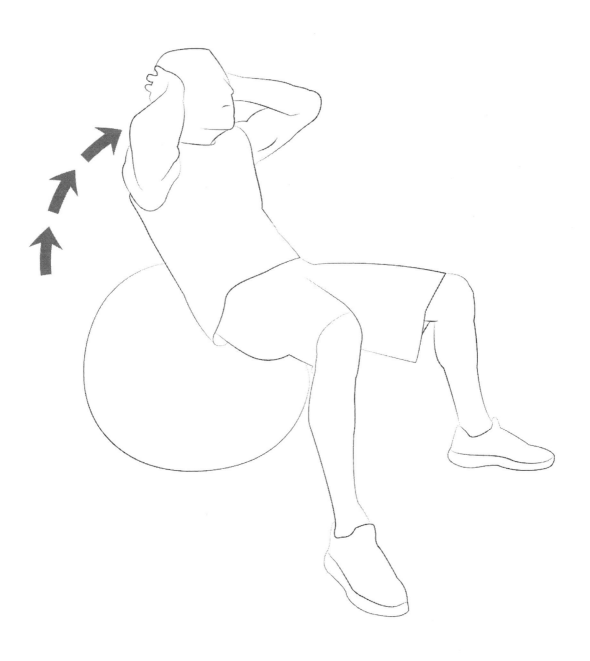

Sit up and bring your head forward and high as possible.

Pause at the top of the sit-up while maintaining continuous tension.

Chapter 12

"Many of life's failures are people who did not realize how close they were to success when they gave up."

- Thomas Edison

Gyms and Personal Trainers

Some people join a gym because they want to change their body and look good. They may be motivated entirely by vanity. Other people join a gym because they want to improve their health and feel better. For most of us, our motivation is some combination of both vanity *and* health. In either case, the formula for achieving your goal and the outcome will be identical. Through my Get Fit, Lean program, you'll lose fat and develop lean muscle, achieving both goals. Therefore, your number one criterion for picking which gym to join and whether or not you decide to hire a personal trainer should be their ability to help you achieve your goals. The gym you join should have all the quality cardio and resistance equipment you need. If you decide to hire a trainer, that trainer should understand that your number one goal is to change your body composition. You need to be confident that this person will help you to lose fat and develop muscle. Don't settle for anything less.

Gyms, fitness centers, and health clubs are not all created equal. They run the gamut from hole-in-the-wall dives to full-on country clubs with immaculate locker rooms and spas that rival the finest resorts. Likewise, personal trainers can range from college kids just out of school who may still be learning the trade, to seasoned professionals with advanced degrees in sports medicine, nutrition and microbiology. To get the maximum benefits of my Get Fit, Lean program, I absolutely recommend joining a well-equipped gym or fitness club in order to have access to all the cardio and resistance training equipment that I discuss and describe. However, whether or not you hire a personal trainer is more of a personal decision. A trainer can certainly be very helpful, especially if serious weight training is new to you or if you are more comfortable having someone to help push and motivate you. You'll have to weigh the variables and decide for yourself.

Selecting the Right Gym for You

In my opinion, the ideal gym is equipped with every conceivable piece of both free weight and resistance training machine. This includes Olympic barbells, several tons of free weights, multiple sets of dumbbells, assortments of benches, seats, weight racks, bars, pulley systems, and other miscellaneous equipment needed for any given exercise. There's a good test to find out how equipped the gym you're considering may be: ask for a tour with the owner, manager or a senior personal trainer. Specifically ask them what your options are for training each of the six major muscle groups. Have the person show you multiple exercise options for back, chest, legs, shoulders, arms (both biceps and triceps) and abs. Additionally, have them also show you different exercise options for each body part using both free weights and weighted resistance machines. Bring with you a list of all the various exercises you'll want to do (the previous chapter of this book is a good one). Make sure there is at least one station where you can perform each exercise on your list.

You may not find the absolute perfect gym, fitness center or health club in your area, but there are certain essential pieces of equipment that all of them should have. I believe there are minimum requirements for complete training. Here are a few of what I consider essential – if they don't have these things, I recommend you keep looking elsewhere:

1. Squat rack
2. Pull up bar
3. Dual cable pulleys
4. Mirrors to view yourself for correct form
5. Enough room to perform dumbbell lunges
6. Enough space and redundant equipment that you don't have to wait in lines during peak workout times (*ie,* morning and after work)
7. Variety of cardio equipment, and multiple pieces of each (treadmill, elliptical trainers, stationary bikes, stair climbers). In addition, all should be well maintained and clean. The cleanliness of a facility can tell you a lot about how well they maintain their equipment. All the equipment in the world won't do you any good if it's broken and poorly maintained.

Cardio machines technology has improved a great deal in recent years, so when touring a facility, be sure to make note of whether they have new equipment, or a few aging examples of older technology. The latter is not a good sign that they are actively improving their facility.

The gym or fitness center should also have enough equipment and space (for cardio AND resistance training) to handle the crowds at peak workout times. Visit a prospective gym or club during the busiest times of day to see how crowded it can become. This is usually just before and after typical weekday working hours, 6:00 am to 9:00 am and 5:00 pm to 8:00 pm. Even if you're lucky enough to have a schedule that allows you to train at off-peak times, you never know. Your schedule or even your job may change. I'd also recommend that you stop and talk to a couple of the members and ask them what they like and don't like about the gym. Another helpful approach is to read reviews on Yelp or other online review sites.

These days it's easy to check out any given business online and find out what people are saying about it.

The last thing to remember is that most gyms and health clubs make you sign a contract for a fixed period of time. Therefore, it's crucial that you shop around and visit multiple facilities to compare what they have – or don't have – before making a commitment. Many of the big chain clubs and gyms have sales staff who are under pressure to make sure you don't walk out the door without signing up. If they tell you their deal is only good for today, then don't believe it. If they want your money, that deal will be there tomorrow or the next day after you've checked out the other facilities. One final tip: many clubs make you pay a sign-up or initiation fee. In many cases these fees are negotiable, so be sure ask what they can do to get the fee down.

Personal Trainers

Before continuing on here regarding my thoughts on personal trainers I want to be clear. I consider these hard working guys and gals part of my fitness family. A good trainer can help you achieve your Get Fit, Lean program goals. Picking the right one for you can add tremendous value. I also have total respect for anyone whose career choice is personal training. Much like nurses, doctors and other health care specialists, they've chosen a job that is dedicated to helping people improve their quality of life. That is an admirable pursuit.

How do you decide whether or not you need a trainer? You need to ask yourself a few questions. First, are you new to resistance training? If you've never picked up a weight or a pair of dumbbells you should consider hiring a personal trainer. How self-motivated are you and how willing are you to learn things on your own? Knowing you've paid for a session in advance is good motivation to get you to the gym. Also, some of us want or need one on one personal demonstration whereas others prefer to figure it out for themselves.

Additionally, are you able to train with the intensity required to get results on your own? Some people may not go for that last rep unless there is someone else pushing them on. If you are the type of person who isn't going to get anything done unless there's someone standing over you saying "don't stop, one more rep" then you might want to hire a personal trainer. You want to make sure you're training with 100% intensity every time you work out. If you choose not to use a personal trainer then, other options are either a reliable training partner or helpful gym regulars.

Also, can you afford it? Hiring a good personal trainer isn't cheap. And many fitness facilities or trainers require you to buy a multiple-session package. I'd recommend that you make sure you can work out once with them to make sure the two of you work well together before investing in a multi-session package. If a trainer won't give you a free initial workout or let you buy a single workout to try them out, then keep looking.

Quite possibly, since you bought this book and are reading it now, you are the self-motivated self-starter type who doesn't need or want to hire a trainer. You may also be the do-it-yourselfer type and you prefer to go it alone. Hiring a personal trainer can help many folks but doing so is not a pre-requisite to success. This book maps out exactly what you need to do and how to go about doing it. Everything you need to know is here if your preference is to do it yourself.

For those of you who do hire a trainer, be very selective. Don't settle for the first trainer that the person who sold you the gym membership or the manager introduces you to. Instead, ask to speak to several potential trainers. Make sure that you feel comfortable with the person you'll eventually be working with. You are the one doing the hiring here so interview as many as you like before making a decision. You're going to spend an hour per session with this person so you'd better be sure that you're both on the same page. Tell them what you are doing and ask how they can help you achieve your goals with this program.

If you already know you're going to hire a trainer before joining a gym, speak to several trainers working out of the different gyms you're considering. This could help you decide which gym to join. The quality and experience of the training staff may influence your gym choice. Think of it and treat it like an interview process. Many of the bigger chain gyms simply need bodies, and therefore employ a lot of trainers on their staff who may or may not have extensive experience or appropriate certifications. In my opinion, you want someone who has both – the knowledge/education as well as experience. I've seen many trainers who have never trained themselves to an elite level, let alone anyone else. I'd recommend that if you're going to hire a trainer, hire someone who can prove they've helped someone like you reach a fitness goal similar to yours.

This leads to what I believe should be a very important criteria in selecting a personal trainer. Has the person that you are considering hiring to help you transform your body and achieve your fitness goals actually done it himself or herself? Does he/she walk the walk? Is this prospective trainer fit, lean, athletic, in great shape, and would you like to emulate this person? If the answer is no, move on and find another trainer. There are several governing bodies that offer online personal training certifications. Anyone can memorize the necessary material and pass an exam. I wouldn't pay any trainer a nickel unless they were in great shape themselves. In my opinion, the only real proof that they know what they're doing is that they've actually done it themselves.

Additionally, if you decide to hire a personal trainer, make one thing perfectly clear. Make sure that he or she understands exactly the results you are looking for before you hire them. The most common complaint that I hear from people who've hired and worked with a personal trainer for months and sometimes years relates to divergent goals. Most people hire a personal trainer because they want to change their body composition. They want to get fit, lean, and look good. Too often the trainer spends the majority of their workout time, typically one-hour sessions, working on other things. Mobility, balance, core exercises and functional movements are all good but you're paying by the hour. Too many people spend countless hours and dollars but in the end up looking the same as when they started.

I've seen another area of concern for years and I continue to see it every day: people working with personal trainers for long periods of time, yet are still significantly over weight. They spend a lot of time and money on a personal trainer when they'd have been much better off hiring a nutritionist instead. Never lose sight of a fundamental principle of the Get Fit, Lean program: if you don't get your nutrition right (*ie,* get your calorie intake under control and eat the right foods), whatever workout you do isn't going to matter a whole lot. The Get Fit,

Lean nutrition plan and workout plan go hand in hand. They are both critical for achieving results.

I'm not saying that personal trainers cannot add value. A good personal trainer can certainly add tremendous value. If you've never stepped foot in a gym, never touched a free weight or worked out on a resistance machine, a trainer can help you quite a lot. If you're apprehensive about getting started or self-conscious or unsure about doing this on your own, then hiring a trainer could also be very helpful. Correct technique, good form and safety should always come first. An experienced trainer can help you learn proper technique. A qualified experienced trainer can make sure you're performing all the exercises I recommend correctly and safely. A good trainer can also teach you some new exercises to mix into your routines.

You will optimize the time and money spent on a trainer by making it clear up front that your primary goal is to shed fat and build lean muscle. The person you hire should understand that focused cardio and intense resistance training to failure is the optimum training method for achieving your goals. Make sure the trainer understands that you're hiring them for their assistance and expertise in learning how to perform traditional weight training muscle isolation exercises and to help you develop lean muscle. Allow the person to teach you how to perform resistance-training exercises correctly and help motivate you to achieve your goals.

Although the trainer may want to show you the latest popular work out style, I recommend that you stick to my plan and not get sidetracked by something else. There are no new training techniques or fad workouts that you've got to do to achieve your goals. Traditional weight training exercises to failure coupled with intense, focused cardio will get you the results you're looking for. Human physiology hasn't changed since the 1950s era of Muscle Beach in Venice, California. There is nothing new under the sun. Getting fit and lean is pretty simple really. You want to build a great physique, get in great shape and be healthy? Eat clean, do cardio and push your weight training to failure. Rest and repeat. That's it.

So choose a good facility that has all the equipment you need to follow my program, and if you think that hiring a trainer will help you succeed, then hire them and make it clear that their job is to help you learn and perform the Get Fit, Lean program.

Chapter 13

"You miss 100% of the shots you don't take."

- Wayne Gretzky

Supplements

Sports nutrition has come a long way since the ancient Greeks began training with barbells in the fifth century BC. We now know much more about how to fuel our bodies for better fitness, health and sports performance. We understand that unlocking our genetic potential is heavily dependent on good nutrition. We also understand the right ratios of macronutrients and micronutrients are required for strength, endurance, recovery, muscle development and general health. We're acutely aware of the many negative health consequences associated with eating processed foods devoid of nutritional value like the processed carbohydrates, flour and sugar.

By now you should be (or preparing to be) following a good nutrition plan and training regime. In this context, consider yourself an athlete. For optimum performance, modern day athletes should be well versed in how to consume the optimal fuel required to unlock their maximum genetic potential. Unfortunately, this may not always be the case. Many people are not getting enough of the nutrients required to fuel and rebuild their body. This is where supplements come in.

Are Supplements Processed Foods?

In a perfect world we would have unlimited access to all varieties of intact whole foods, all of the time. If this were the case, we'd be able to get all the nutrients our bodies require from whole food sources alone. Unfortunately, in practice few if any of us have unlimited access to intact whole foods all of the time, due to reasons such as availability, seasonality, convenience and location, to name a few. Low nutrient density in much of our nation's soil also results in poor quality crops. Nutritional supplements can and should fill the void.

A fair amount of my nutrition plan argues against consuming processed foods. But let me be clear in explaining that not all processed foods are created equal, and therefore they should not all be vilified. Most processed foods are indeed bad for you, but in the case of certain nutritional supplements, they may be exactly what you need. Let me explain; food-like products like white sugar and refined flour are made using a process that degrades or destroys the nutritional value of what was previously a whole food. Conversely, when supplements such as whey protein isolate and glutamine are made, the reverse occurs. Nutritional value is instead extracted from a whole food. The difference between the two is in the nutritional content of the final product. When a whole grain is processed to create refined flour, most if not all of the nutritional value is either destroyed or stripped away. However, in the case of whey protein isolate, a valuable muscle building supplement, the nutritional value is isolated via making cheese from milk. The whey protein is then extracted, packaged and made available to you in order to supplement your predominately intact whole food meal plan.

When and Why Should You Consider Taking Supplements?

Supplements are by definition substances added to complete something, make up for a deficiency, or extend or strengthen the whole. In terms of eating right, intact whole foods should be your first choice. The majority of your calories should come from whole foods. However, it's often difficult to get enough of certain nutrients by relying solely on whole food sources. Protein is an excellent example of this. The Get Fit, Lean nutrition plan calls for eating six times a day, and each one of those meals or snacks includes a protein. It can be hard to rely on whole foods alone to consume enough protein in a day. The reality is that eating six portions of lean protein a day (for example, chicken breast) requires a heck of a lot of food preparation, and can also become very monotonous. Therefore, I recommend that you consider getting 2 or even 3 of your daily protein servings from a high quality protein supplement. In fact, a protein shake may be your best choice just after training.

Intense exercise breaks down muscle and protein supplements repair and build muscle. Whey protein negotiates through the stomach quickly and then is rapidly absorbed in the intestine.[53] Protein synthesis levels are heightened after a workout.[54] Therefore, because whey is digested and absorbed very quickly, I recommend taking a whey protein supplement within twenty minutes of your resistance training everyday. Conversely, casein protein is absorbed slowly so should be taken before going to bed at night in order to supply a steady supply of muscle repairing protein as you sleep.

Additionally, some supplements can be taken to ensure we are meeting all of our body's micronutrient needs. As much as our intentions are good and we try our best to eat healthy foods containing the right ratios of macronutrients that are also rich in micronutrients, we can still fall short of what our bodies actually need - especially when engaged in a high-intensity exercise and cardio program that taxes your body on a daily basis. Therefore, I recommend that you consider taking a high quality multi-vitamin and mineral supplement taken together with an essential omega fatty acid supplement to ensure that you're getting all your micronutrients every day.

Some supplements help your body tolerate intense exercise longer and aid in your recovery and the building of lean muscle. Our bodies naturally make and store certain nutrients in very small quantities. We can quickly deplete these small stores during intense exercise. Creatine is a good example of a micronutrient that we all store naturally in our muscle cells in very small quantities.

Let's return for a moment to how evolution has shaped our design for survival. Humans are very well adapted for short burst of intense physical activity. Like most other animals, we have special energy stores for either running after food or running away to avoid becoming food. High intensity training, especially weight training, requires repeated short bursts of energy. Weight training for extended periods of time depletes our stores of certain micronutrients like glutamine and creatine. Creatine helps supply energy to muscle cells but our bodies manufacture and store it in very small quantities. Glutamine is an amino acid that helps rebuild muscle after heavy training. I believe that creatine and glutamine are useful supplements that can help extend or top off your body's naturally occurring stores of these valuable micronutrients.

Depending on your long-term fitness goals and your budget, you may not want to or be able to buy all the supplements I recommend. At a minimum I strongly encourage you to take a quality multi-vitamin and mineral supplement along with an omega fatty acid supplement. I'll explain why in a couple of pages.

Quality

Like most consumer products, you get what you pay for. Most of the time this may seem obvious, however in the case of supplements it may not be. Most people understand and agree that a cheap, low-quality cut of steak and a filet mignon are two very different things. However, when it comes to most supplements, quality differences are not so apparent. Lower quality supplements may contain sugar, sweeteners, artificial flavors, unknown filler additives, and can taste great. In addition, because they are often in powder form, many of the supplements look the same and so differences in quality may not be obvious. There can however be significant differences in quality between supplement manufacturers even if the macronutrients seem comparable.

Unfortunately, in the US, the Food and Drug Administration regulates dietary supplements under a different set of regulations than those covering "conventional" food and drug products. Supplement manufacturers are not required to register their products with the FDA or get FDA approval before producing or selling their products. Supplement manufacturers are instead responsible for their own quality control and the accuracy of their label information. As a result of this lack of regulation, the raw materials used in some supplements may not be from the best sources, the manufacturing facility may not be the cleanest and the label may not even represent what's actually in the supplement.

One way to help identify high quality supplements is by looking for an NSF (National Sanitation Foundation), the public health and safety organization and GMP (Good Manufacturing Practices) inspection stamp on the product's label. Both the NSF and GMP are recognized 3rd party product testing organizations that certify that the manufacturing process meets their standards (although it's important to note that neither test to confirm that what is printed on the label is actually what is in the product). Some supplement manufactures have their own internal quality control department or hire a third party in order to stamp a QIG (Quality Ingredients Guarantee) on the label. The bottom line is that you'll need to be a smart consumer, read labels, do some research on the manufacturer, and try to read 3rd party product reviews (from a lab, not a forum) before buying any supplements. Like any consumer product, there are low and high quality supplements. I recommend that you stick with the highest quality supplements that you're able to buy.

Nutritional supplements support your good health. To me, they're worth spending money on. I'm betting most people spend money on more things that are *not* good for them. Trade some bad habits in for some good ones. For example, if you buy a Starbuck's venti mocha cappuccino every day, trade it for a grande coffee of the day. You'll be getting no sugar, and you'll be saving nearly 2 to 3 bucks a day. Use that new-found money on something healthy like your supplements.

Recommended Supplements

As I mentioned, you may or may not want to buy these or you may not be able to afford them all, but if you can, I'd recommend the following. I try to avoid recommending specific brands; there are many out there and I'd encourage you to spend some time researching them so that you have the information you need to choose the one that fits your needs, budget, and is of the best quality you can afford.

Multi-Vitamin and Minerals

A daily multi-vitamin and mineral supplement will ensure that you're getting all of your essential micronutrients and antioxidants. These are not all created equal. What you're looking for is bioavailability. Are the vitamins and minerals in a form that your body can utilize or will they pass right through you? You can answer this question by reading independent product reviews so do your research and buy the highest quality you can afford.[55] It may be time to upgrade from the Flintstone Chewables.

Omega 3-6-9 Fatty Acids

Take this supplement daily along with your multi-vitamin and minerals for improved absorption of your vitamins. Omega 3-6-9 fatty acids support brain, eye, and cognitive functions. They also help lipid (fat) metabolism, cardiovascular health, joint function, immune function, and skin health. They also play a vital role in many cellular and metabolic processes.

Whey Protein Isolate

Whey protein isolate has a high rate of digestion so is best taken immediately after intense resistance training. It is 90% protein by weight and contains high levels of all the essential amino acids and branched-chain amino acids. Our bodies use amino acids (the building blocks of protein) to aid in muscle recovery and muscle growth.

Casein Protein

I recommend that you take a casein-based protein supplement as your last meal before going to bed, because its slow rate of digestion provides a sustained release of amino acids while you sleep.

Both casein and whey proteins are made from milk, where they naturally occur. For those who are lactose sensitive or intolerant, you may experience bloating or other digestive discomfort. If this is the case, you will need to try a protein supplement that is not milk-based. Alternative protein supplements are derived from egg white, beef or plant-based proteins.

Protein Bars vs Protein Powder

Just because your favorite gym, health club or fitness center sells protein and nutrition bars doesn't mean that they're something you should be eating. Many of these so called nutrition bars are little more than candy bars with some whey protein added. After a hard workout you understandably feel famished and can't wait to treat yourself with something good to eat. Besides, you should be consuming some sort of protein in the 20-30 minute window following a workout as this is a critical time for replenishing your body and rebuilding lean muscle. On your way out of the gym you might pass by a display of supplements for sale, including protein and nutrition bars. The labels boast 20, 25 or 30 grams of protein per bar and some might even have a reasonable macronutrient profile, seemingly exactly what you need. They also come in a wide variety of tempting flavors like chocolate chip, cookies and cream, strawberry cheesecake and many other delicious sounding options. You think, this is exactly what I need to replenish my starving muscles. Not necessarily.

I see a lot of people stop to buy some kind of bar on their way out of the gym. As convenient and satisfying as these may be, you can make much better choices. Pre-packaged protein and nutrition bars have either artificial sweeteners or added sugar and a lot of filler carbohydrates in order to physically hold them together. The filler carbohydrates are not the kind of whole food carbohydrates you should be eating. Additionally, like any other pre-packaged food-like product, they're loaded with chemical preservatives because they've got to have a shelf life.

By comparison, a high quality protein powder mixed with water is a far better post-workout choice. Protein powder doesn't need to be held together in a bar-like shape, so it has no filler carbohydrates. Liquid protein is also more readily available than solid protein when it comes to fueling your hungry muscles.[56] Liquid protein delivers amino acids, the building blocks of protein, to your blood stream faster than solid proteins.[57] This is especially important during that critical 20 to

30 minute window to feed your muscle tissue that immediately follows a hard workout.

So my advice is to plan ahead, add a couple of scoops of your favorite protein powder in a shaker bottle and toss it in your gym bag. After your workout just add cold water, shake it up, and you've got a great source of pure protein to drink without any unnecessary carbs. Unless there are no other options and you're in a pinch, I don't recommend eating pre-packaged bars. A much better source of post workout protein is a high quality powder supplement drink that you mix yourself. You can make much better use of the available calories from carbohydrates in your nutrition plan than the inherent filler carbohydrates in pre-packaged bars.

Glutamine

Glutamine is not an essential amino acid but can become conditionally essential in certain situations like intense athletic training. Glutamine aids in muscle recovery and is good for your general health. It helps fortify your immune system and aids in digestion. Because our muscle cells have limited absorption capacity, it's recommended that you don't take creatine and glutamine together. I mix my glutamine in my casein protein shake taken at the end of the day.

Creatine

Creatine is a naturally occurring micronutrient found mostly in red meat. It's an organic acid that our bodies store predominately in skeletal muscle. Creatine is a combination of three different amino acids; glycine, arginine, and methionine. Creatine increases your body's adenine tri-phosphate (ATP) stores. ATP is your body's energy source for nearly every body function, including muscle contraction. Your body oxidizes carbohydrates, protein or fat in order to produce ATP.

Creatine has been shown in studies to increase strength and lean muscle mass during high-intensity, short-duration exercise, such as weight lifting thus im-proving our response to resistance training.[58] I've found that creatine works very well when taken as directed. I've experienced significant strength and muscle development gains using creatine. It's best taken just before and just after your resistance training. As I mentioned previously, it's recommended that you don't take creatine and glutamine at the same time, because our muscle cells have limited absorption capacity. More efficient absorption of each is achieved by taking them separately (which is why I take my glutamine just before bed).

Creatine is sold in several forms, but creatine monohydrate is my preference. Although some people report significant strength gains (myself included), other people experience uncomfortable stomach issues like gas and bloating. If you are one of those people who do not tolerate creatine, don't worry. It's by no means necessary for my Get Fit, Lean program. I simply recommend it as an adjunct for building muscle and performance.

Caffeine

Caffeine is my go-to pre-workout supplement of choice. Caffeine increases your metabolic rate and improves cognitive function, which helps aid weight loss by making your cardio training more effective. Research has shown that caffeine improves athletic performance and through antagonizing the neurotransmitter adenosine, which tells the brain when we are tired, alleviates fatigue.[59] Caffeine also improves alertness, attention, focus and concentration. There is also evidence that caffeine is associated with improved memory and cognitive function. For these reasons, I recommend caffeine as an effective energy booster.

Although I recommend caffeine, it may not be for everyone. There are side effects from too much caffeine, and as a result I'd recommend that you control your intake. Too much caffeine can increase blood pressure and heart rate, and can cause shakiness or tremors. Caffeine taken late in the day may also cause sleep problems like insomnia. Moderate caffeine consumption is considered between 200 and 300 mg per day or about two to four cups of coffee a day. Between 500 and 600 mg of caffeine per day or more than four cups per day is considered heavy consumption. The caffeine content of a typical 12 oz cola can range from 40 to 70 mg, depending on the specific product. A 12 to 16 oz cup of coffee-house coffee from your favorite café chain can contain between 70 to 250 mg of caffeine, and popular energy drinks can contain over 300 mg of caffeine in a single can. Unfortunately, the FDA does not require quantitative caffeine labeling – the bare minimum we need to make informed choices of appropriate doses.[60] Consume these highly caffeinated products judiciously.

Daily caffeine drinkers seem to be less likely to experience adverse effects but everyone is affected differently. High doses can cause anxiety or in extreme cases hallucinations. Limit your caffeine consumption to early morning and/or just before working out. I believe caffeine consumption can help a great deal in burning calories, losing weight and getting through intense training sessions, but you've got to be the judge of whether it's a good supplement for you, and how much is appropriate.

So what are the optimal sources of caffeine? Well, many people mistakenly think that caffeine and coffee are synonymous. However, caffeine and coffee is *not* the same thing. It's true that many people use coffee as a delivery mechanism for caffeine – including me. I'm a coffee lover. Having a warm cup of coffee is part of my morning routine. I can't imagine not drinking a warm cup of coffee in the morning. However, I try to limit my coffee consumption to no more than two cups a day.

If coffee is not your cup of tea, well, tea is also a good source of caffeine. By volume, tea averages about half the caffeine of coffee. Tea is cleansing as it contains catechins, which are natural antioxidants. The catechin concentrations are highest in white and green teas with less occurring in black teas.

Many people use various popular bottled pre-workout drinks and energy drinks as their caffeine delivery systems. These are quite popular, but often contain sugar or sweeteners as well as other added ingredients that may not be optimal for your nutrition plan. Along with caffeine, most energy drinks also add some "proprietary blend" of thermogenic herbs, meaning the manufacturer is not going to tell you what's in it. For this reason, I recommend trying to find clean caffeine sources. By clean I mean caffeine sources with no sugar or artificial sweeteners added. I've found one energy drink that I consider clean, *hi*ball ENERGY*. I appreciate that the manufacturer lists the ingredients of their proprietary formula on the product's label. The unsweetened version contains zero calories, 160 mg of caffeine, 50 mg of guarana, and 50 mg of ginseng. Taking caffeine pills is always an alternative to any type of caffeinated drink as well as a good way to know exactly how much caffeine your consuming but personally I prefer coffee, tea, and my clean caffeine source.

Chapter 14

"It always seems impossible until it's done."

- Nelson Mandela

Let's Get Going

You're now armed with all the tools you need to succeed in following my Get Fit, Lean program. You understand how to put all three critical components of my program into action. You'll combine good nutrition, cardio exercise and resistance training to transform your body composition. If you haven't already done so, it's time now to draw a line in the sand and mark a date on the calendar. I recommend starting my program on a Monday so that you can kick your week off strong and get into your new scheduled routine. Choose a target goal weight, commit yourself, and follow my program for 12 weeks.

Follow-Through, Staying the Course

Let's fast forward three months to your first milestone. You stayed on your nutrition plan, you worked your butt off in the gym, you reached your weight loss goal and you reshaped your body composition. You're looking good. Congratulations! Well done. You deserve a well-earned reward. It's party time! Pop the cork on some good bubbly, belly up to your favorite buffet brunch, take a week off the gym and put it all back on. Right?

Please no. Stop and think about how hard you worked to get to where you are now. Please take it from me, the cheat meal(s) you've dreamed about for months can quickly become a cheat week and snowball out of control into ten to twenty unwanted pounds in no time at all. Over indulgent cheat meals are a slippery slope. Admittedly, my weight loss has yo-yoed a few times and I've learned some hard lessons along the way. Immediately following my first physique competition I spun a little out of control gaining 10 pounds in a weekend and 20 pounds in a few weeks. Avoiding the yo-yo and maintaining your hard won new physique may be more difficult than doing the actual body transformation itself.

Plan to Succeed

In mid-journey, when you're locked into a structured routine of good nutrition and exercise, it's easier to stay on the right track. When your meal plan and workout schedules are regimented, all you've got to do is follow the script. When I'm working towards a specific weight goal and a hard date on the calendar, I plan exactly what and how much I'm going to eat every day. I also plan exactly how many calories I'm going to burn doing cardio every day. After I start to see real results, I also seem to instinctively crank up the weight training intensity. Using an online calorie counter I plan my meal diary either the night before or every morning. After that I just follow the program, log my new improved weight each morning and watch by body composition change. Psychologically, it feels great to see real progress in the mirror. There's a great deal of satisfaction in staying on track and seeing real tangible results happening right before your eyes.

In fact, most of us are goal oriented. Marking a day on the calendar and setting a hard and fast goal is a great way to force the issue when striving to achieve any goal.

Our probability of success improves dramatically when we set goals. The idea that you're now committed to achieving something is a powerful motivator. Another hint that will help ensure success is don't keep your transformation a secret. Tell as many people close to you as possible and you'll see them become your biggest fans. Your friends, family, and colleagues at work asking you how it's going will provide additional motivation throughout your transformation. All of these people will become part of your support network along the way.

Set a Maintenance Plan

As I mentioned, achieving your goal may be less difficult than maintaining the result. With no goal on the horizon, it's easy to lose your inspiration. I've experienced this post competition. Taking your body fat down below 7% is more extreme than most people who follow my program will do. However, everyone will wrestle with the same demons. After 12 weeks of a strict nutrition plan, the lure of short-term gratification from decadent foods can be a powerful temptation. You need a long-term maintenance plan in hand and ready to implement immediately following your 12 week transformation. Don't consider yourself "done", because you should never be done. Fitness and health is a lifelong endeavor. Remember, it's a lifestyle, not a diet.

Start you maintenance plan the same way you started your original transformation: choose a date on the calendar 12 weeks out and then carve that date in stone. Give yourself a more modest goal this time perhaps losing or gaining as little as one to two pounds. Resolve and determination to achieve your new goal by that future date is a large part of what will keep you on track.

Managing the Occasional Cheat Meal

It's only natural that once your original goal is reached you'd want to reward yourself. You indeed deserve a reward. I'd be lying if I claimed that my reward wasn't some decadent food I'd avoided for three months. A cheat meal is ok. You can and should enjoy some limited forbidden fruit without completely going off the rails.

Pick a day, invite someone close to you or a group of friends and make it a special occasion. I believe that the occasional decadent meal is good for the soul. The trick is not to make every meal a cheat meal for an entire day, weekend or an entire week. I've found a couple of practical ideas that help keep me from slipping off track. They should work for you too.

First, don't sit down to your cheat meal when you've eaten very little that day. If you're feeling like you're absolutely starving to death you will more likely gorge. Instead, fill up on healthy foods early on the day of your planned cheat meal. If you're going to blow out your calories on a day then do it with mostly good healthy calories. Think of it as pre-emptive damage control. If, when you tuck into that large pizza or plate of pasta you've been dying for, you've already had a chicken breast and asparagus a few hours before, you'll be much less likely to go too far off the rails by eating copious amounts of junk calories.

Second, continue to log your meals in your online food diary after you've completed your 12-week transformation. I've found this extremely helpful in not slipping up to bad. Religiously logging that 5,000 calorie pizza in your food diary after 3 months of 1,600 to 2,600 calories a day can have a dramatic psychological affect. Just seeing that huge calorie number in your food diary may be enough to curb future cheat meals. Not logging your meals in your food diary is along the lines of out of site out of mind. For example, I've been away on vacation enjoying local cuisine for a few days and not bothered to log anything I ate. It's amazing how fast good intentions can all go out the window. Once you've lost track of how many calories you've eaten, it's easy to lose all control. You can quickly become a victim of the "I'm already dirty" syndrome. Don't allow yourself the opportunity to fall into the very dangerous mindset of "at this point it just doesn't matter anymore."

Maintenance: A Reverse Plan

As much as I hate to use the word "diet," I'll make this one exception. I'm able to rationalize doing so only because what I'm about to describe is commonly referred to as "reverse dieting." Diet in this case may indeed be the most suitable word because it is in fact temporary. You may gain back a pound or two but as long as it's for the purpose of establishing your new calorie baseline that's ok.

Let's say for example that you're a 35-year-old woman who started my program weighing 165 pounds and after 12 weeks reached your goal weight of 130 pounds goal weight. Or you may be a 45-year-old man whose beginning weight was 230 pounds and now after 12 weeks you weigh 180 pounds. During the course of your 12-week transformations, you were able to lose 2 to 4 pounds per week by staying in calorie deficit. Your daily calorie intakes were 1600 and 2300 calories respectively. Now that you've reached your goal weight you no longer want to stay in calorie deficit but rather eat just enough to remain calorie neutral. You need to find the right amount of calories to both consume and burn in order to maintain what you've achieved. You need to establish a new daily calorie baseline that enables you to maintain your new weight and body composition.

Employ the same methodology you used to find the daily calorie total that put you in calorie deficit. First, use your online calorie counter's algorithm, then tweak it if necessary using a little trial and error. You'll find a new calorie intake that enables you to maintain your new and improved current weight. The calorie counter's algorithm is imperfect because it relies on assumptions that may or may not be completely accurate. As previously discussed, the algorithm is generic and everyone's biochemistry is a little different, but nevertheless it's going to be a good starting point. If you do need to make adjustments as you go, then make incremental small ones.

If you're happy with your new weight and body composition then you can slowly increase your calories so that you're no longer in calorie deficit but rather calorie neutral. Begin by increasing your daily calorie intake by just one to two hundred calories a day. Go from 1600 to 1700 or 2300 to 2500 calories respectively. Continue to log your meals every day and record your weight every morning. If you begin gaining or losing more weight than you intended, slightly re-adjust your total daily calorie consumption. What will also help you transition from calorie deficit to lifetime maintenance is to mark another date of the calendar. Set a maintenance goal weight. Choose a date 12 weeks out, starting from when you reached your initial transformation goal weight and make that your new goal.

Even if it's exactly the same weight you are now, maintaining exactly the same weight you are now is a noteworthy goal and a challenge in itself. Setting that new goal will give you a physiological advantage. The same strategy that helped get you to where you are now can be employed to help you maintain your new weight, your new body composition and your new healthy lifestyle.

Fit and Lean for Life

Unlike your fitness and nutrition journey, this book must come to an end. I've thought long and hard about how to close this read. Some Zen like motivational or inspirational message always seemed most appropriate but also feels too obvious and a bit canned.

The best motivation is that which comes from within *you*. Once you've reached your initial goals, continue to tap into the same inner strength that helped get you there in the first place. You'll be tempted by bad food choices the rest of your life. Every time you sit down in a restaurant and open a menu, go to a dinner party, drive past a freeway off ramp or walk past the junk food aisle (almost every aisle, unfortunately) in the grocery store you'll have to tap into your inner strength. Be strong and choose long-term health over short-term gratification. It's not always going to be easy; if it were easy then everybody would be in great shape.

Every morning when you step on your bathroom scale or check yourself out in a mirror months and years from now, you'll take pride in what you've achieved. Also take pride in your steadfast resolve that has enabled you maintain the new fit you. Once you've truly embraced the health and fitness lifestyle you'll reap the rewards daily. Feeling and looking great can never be overvalued. You cannot put a price tag on good health. Every morning when you wake up to start your day take a moment to feel your flat stomach and take gratification in your physical wellbeing. Go about your day with self-confidence and the quiet satisfaction that you're one of an exceptional minority. You're now a member of an elite club. You're in great shape. Friends, family, colleagues and everyone you interact with throughout the day will take notice of your fit physique, not to mention your improved self-esteem. Take pride in what you've accomplished and hold yourself up as an example that inspires others to follow in your footsteps. You may be surprised by just how inspiring you can be.

You're now armed with everything you need to know to succeed in your transformation. You know good nutrition, the importance of cardio, and resistance training. Your new and improved you is waiting, so let's get going! It's all here for you in this book, you just need to take that first step and make it happen. Get Fit, Lean and take pride in the healthy new you.

Appendix A

Twelve-Week Body Transformation Contest Essay

May 31, 2009

Earlier this year I went to see my doctor for what I thought would be a routine physical. Back in the fall I had been laid off from my job, and I knew it was probably a good idea to get a physical while I still had health insurance. I am 43 years old, have not gone for a checkup in many years and had really let myself go physically—often indulging in decadent meals and too much beer—but I still believed the visit with my doctor would be completely uneventful. I thought I was in good health, so I expected nothing more than an uneventful checkup ending with the doctor sending me on my way.

As it turned out, I was wrong. Preliminary tests showed I had potentially serious problems with my colon, my prostate, and my heart. My doctor sent me to three different specialists who could perform additional tests. Over the next few weeks I endured several hospital visits, a battery of medical tests, and many sleepless nights where I was consumed with anxiety about my health. At first I was most worried that test results would confirm I had colon or prostate cancer, but then I met with a cardiologist who worried me further by telling me he thought I had blockage in my arteries. He sent me for a heart catheter—a nasty, invasive procedure that left me barely able to walk for the next two weeks.

Throughout this time I was an emotional wreck. I ate every meal as if it was my last—letting myself pig out on all of my favorite foods. I became a regular at local cheeseburger and Tex-Mex restaurants. My mid-section ballooned, and for the first time in my life I weighed over 210 pounds. In the end, I had been worrying for nothing—all of my test results came back negative. I had just wasted a month of my life with doctor's appointments, probes, procedures, and sleepless nights, and all I had to show for it was the weight I had gained.

With a clearer head on my shoulders, I became disgusted with what I saw when I looked in the mirror. Over the years I had gradually replaced the athletic physique I maintained in college with that of an out of shape middle-aged man. I decided I had to make a real change.

After all of my medical tests came back normal, I felt like I had dodged a bullet. Three bullets, even. I knew I was lucky to have my health and that I needed to start making the most of it. I had a wife and two kids—a six-year-old girl and an eight-year-old boy—who are very active in sports, and I knew I wanted to be able to keep up with them in any sport they chose. I started practicing some eating discipline, and working hard in the gym. I felt like I had the energy I had at 18. My morning cardio workout kick-started my metabolism, which meant that while most of my co-workers at my new job headed straight for the coffee machine each morning, I'm was alert and ready to tackle the day. I found that my frequent healthy, high protein, high fat, low carbohydrate meals gave me continuous energy throughout the day. Instead of the post-lunch food comas I had gotten used to fighting, I felt energized and productive all day long. I no longer spent my weekends sleeping in and taking afternoon naps. Instead I sprang from bed in the morning and had the energy to go for bike rides or run around playing with my kids for as long as they wanted.

People now ask me how I'm able to wake up so early every day to get in my cardio and resistance training routine before work. Some people think I'm suffering and enduring some sort of hardship working out so much. What I tell them is that I get my inspiration from people who have endured *real* suffering and hardship. For instance, I think of how Navy SEAL Marcus Luttrell survived a brutal firefight with Taliban fighters outnumbering him 100 to 1 in the mountains of Afghanistan. By comparison, there are no bad guys firing machine guns at me on my spin bike in the morning. There are also the countless displaced people from conflicts around the globe who survive months even years in refugee camps without adequate food or clean water. These folks don't have chocolate protein shakes at their ready disposal. My inspiration is all around us. I consider my ability to work out, eat healthy foods, and stay fit a privilege, not a hardship. My transformation motivated me to be the best father, the best employee and best person I could be—all while getting into the best shape of my life.

Sincerely,

JD

Appendix B

Sample Resistance Training Routines

Heavy Week

Choose three exercises and do three sets of each exercise for a total of nine sets. Using trial and error, find a weight whereby you fail at between 8 to 12 reps then require assistance for the last 2 reps (forced reps). Push each set to failure.

Super Set Week

Choose two combinations of two exercises each for each combination. Do three sets of each two exercise combination without resting between exercises within the super set. In total, you'll do twelve sets. Find a weight for each exercise whereby you fail at between 20 and 30 reps. Always do a warm up set first using light weights (which doesn't count as a "real set").

Six-Day Split (Preferred)

Day 1, Back

- Warm up with pull-ups or light lat pull downs
- Pull-ups, use weighted pull-ups if you're able
- Hammer strength rows (or machine rows)
- Wide grip pull-downs, 3 sets of 8 to 12 reps to failure
- Seated narrow grip cable rows, 3 sets of 8 to 12 reps to failure
- Dumbbell shrugs
- T-bar Rows, either free weight or a T-bar machine
- Farmer's walk (carry a dumbbell in each hand and walk the length of your fitness area up and back, or up and down stairs if your gym has 2 floors)

Day 2, Chest

- Warm up with light bench press or dumbbell press
- Bench press or inclined bench press
- Dumbbell press or inclined dumbbell press
- Inclined cable cross-overs
- Pec deck
- Push-ups
- TRX bodyweight push-ups

Day 3, Legs and Glutes

- Warm up with light squats or dumbbell lunges
- Squats
- Deadlifts
- Dumbbell lunges
- Leg press
- Leg extensions
- Cable kick-backs
- Calf raises
- Stiff-legged dead lifts

Day 4, Shoulders
- Seated dumbbell press
- Dumbbell raises, either to the front or the side
- Upright rows
- Rear deltoid cable rows

Day 5, Arms (Biceps and Triceps)
- Straight bar curls (standing)
- Seated dumbbell curls
- Seated hammer curls
- Preacher curls using EZ curl bar
- Tricep push-downs
- Nose busters (triceps extensions lying on flat bench)
- Dips
- Narrow grip bench press

Day 6, Abs
- TRX crunches from plank
- TRX pike crunches from plank
- Hanging leg raises
- Stability ball sit-ups

Day 7, Rest and Recovery

Five-Day Split (Combine Shoulders and Abs)

Day 1, Back
- Warm up with pull-ups or light lat pull downs
- Pull-ups, use weighted pull-ups if you're able
- Hammer strength rows (or machine rows)
- Wide grip pull-downs, 3 sets of 8 to 12 reps to failure

- Seated narrow grip cable rows, 3 sets of 8 to 12 reps to failure
- Dumbbell shrugs
- T-bar Rows, either free weight or a T-bar machine
- Farmer's walk (carry a dumbbell in each hand and walk the length of your fitness area up and back, or up and down stairs if your gym has 2 floors)

Day 2, Chest
- Warm up with light bench press or dumbbell press
- Bench press or inclined bench press
- Dumbbell press or inclined dumbbell press
- Inclined cable cross-overs
- Pec deck
- Push-ups
- TRX bodyweight push-ups

Day 3, Legs and Glutes
- Warm up with light squats or dumbbell lunges
- Squats
- Deadlifts
- Dumbbell lunges
- Leg press
- Leg extensions
- Cable kick-backs
- Calf raises
- Stiff-legged dead lifts

Day 4, Rest and Recovery
- Cardio training only

Day 5, Shoulders and Abs
- Seated dumbbell press
- Upright rows

- Rear deltoid cable rows
- TRX crunches from plank
- TRX pike crunches from plank
- Hanging leg raises

Day 6, Arms (Biceps and Triceps)

- Straight bar curls (standing)
- Seated dumbbell curls
- Seated hammer curls
- Preacher curls using EZ curl bar
- Tricep push-downs
- Nose busters (triceps extensions lying on flat bench)
- Dips
- Narrow grip bench press

Day 7, Rest and Recovery

Four-Day Split (Combine Back and Chest)

Day 1, Back and Chest

- Warm up with pull-ups or light lat pull downs
- Pull-ups, use weighted pull-ups if you're able
- Hammer strength rows (or machine rows)
- Seated narrow grip cable rows, 3 sets of 8 to 12 reps to failure
- Dumbbell shrugs
- Farmer's walk (carry a dumbbell in each hand and walk the length of your fitness area up and back, or up and down stairs if your gym has 2 floors)
- Warm up with light bench press or dumbbell press
- Bench press or inclined bench press
- Dumbbell press or inclined dumbbell press
- Inclined cable cross-overs
- Push-ups

Day 2, Rest and Recovery
- Cardio training only

Day 3, Legs and Glutes
- Warm up with light squats or dumbbell lunges
- Squats
- Deadlifts
- Dumbbell lunges
- Leg press
- Leg extensions
- Cable kick-backs
- Calf raises
- Stiff-legged dead lifts

Day 4, Rest and Recovery
- Cardio training only

Day 5, Shoulders and Abs
- Seated dumbbell press
- Upright rows
- Rear deltoid cable rows
- TRX crunches from plank
- TRX pike crunches from plank
- Hanging leg raises

Day 6, Arms (Biceps and Triceps)
- Straight bar curls (standing)
- Seated dumbbell curls
- Seated hammer curls
- Preacher curls using EZ curl bar
- Tricep push-downs
- Nose busters (triceps extensions lying on flat bench)

- Dips
- Narrow grip bench press

Day 7, Rest and Recovery

Three-Day Split (Combine Legs and Shoulders Then Also Combine Abs, Biceps, and Triceps)

Day 1, Back and Chest
- Warm up with pull-ups or light lat pull downs
- Pull-ups, use weighted pull-ups if you're able
- Hammer strength rows (or machine rows)
- Seated narrow grip cable rows, 3 sets of 8 to 12 reps to failure
- Dumbbell shrugs
- Farmer's walk (carry a dumbbell in each hand and walk the length of your fitness area up and back, or up and down stairs if your gym has 2 floors)
- Warm up with light bench press or dumbbell press
- Bench press or inclined bench press
- Dumbbell press or inclined dumbbell press
- Inclined cable cross-overs
- Push-ups

Day 2, Rest and Recovery
- Cardio training only

Day 3, Legs, Glutes, and Shoulders
- Warm up with light squats or dumbbell lunges
- Squats
- Deadlifts
- Dumbbell lunges
- Leg press
- Leg extensions

- Cable kick-backs
- Calf raises
- Stiff-legged dead lifts
- Seated dumbbell press
- Upright rows
- Rear deltoid cable rows

Day 4, Rest and Recovery
- Cardio training only

Day 5, Rest and Recovery

Day 6, Biceps, Triceps, and Abs
- Straight bar curls (standing)
- Seated dumbbell curls
- Seated hammer curls
- Preacher curls using EZ curl bar
- Tricep push-downs
- Nose busters (triceps extensions lying on flat bench)
- Dips
- Narrow grip bench press
- TRX crunches from plank
- TRX pike crunches from plank
- Hanging leg raises

Day 7, Rest and Recovery

Appendix C

Program Outline

Get Fit, Lean and Keep your Day Job
1. Nutrition
    a. Create an online calorie counter account (I recommend myfitnesspal.com, and you can use the online tool or the app or both)
    b. Establish Target 12-week weight goal
    c. Determine total allowed calories
    d. Put yourself in calorie deficit
    e. Log all calories consumed
    f. Manually input your macronutrient ratios
        2. 45% protein, 35% fat and 20% carbohydrates
    g. Eat intact whole foods
        1. Eat NO refined carbohydrates
        2. No sugar, No flour
2. Cardio Training
    a. Choose cardio exercises you're comfortable with
    b. Establish your target heart rate in bpm
    c. Do 30 to 60 minutes 5 to 7 days per week

    d. Mix up your cardio exercises

    e. Log your calories burned as calorie credits

3. Resistance Training

    a. Choose the split that fits your schedule

    b. Train each muscle once a week

    c. Train with intensity and focus to failure

    d. Alternate heavy and light weeks

    e. Practice muscle confusion

Acknowledgments

Five years ago, when I decided to write a transformation guide, I hade no idea of the scale of the project I was getting myself into. The completion of this book would not have been possible without the help and support of many people who were very generous with their time. I'd like to thank those friends who were kind enough to spend time proofreading drafts of my manuscript and then offer constructive feedback. Without their input, this book would not have been possible.

Nadine Manfredi, Jim Ferrill, Brad Schaeffer, Jason Hanna, Dominic Magnabosco, Matt Cooper, Sajjad Khan, Chuck Carlton, Jim Campbell, Anthony Parvin, Faris Griffin, and Zianah Griffin gave me valuable suggestions along the way. I am grateful to all of you.

Special thanks goes to Steve Welch, editor extraordinaire. Steve, always the consummate professional and brilliant writer, helped me transform a rough manuscript into a polished transformation guide. Steve completely immersed himself into my book project, reading, re-reading and contributing valuable advice all along the way. I don't think I could have completed this without your help. Thank you, Steve.

References

[1] World Health Organization, "Obesity and Overweight Fact Sheet," www.who.int, March 2013

[2] DJ Frenk, "A Global Look at Rising Obesity Rates," Harvard School of Public Health, www.hsph.harvard.edu

[3] Robert H. Lustig, M.D., <u>Fat Chance: Beating the Odds Against Sugar, Processed Food, Obesity, and Disease</u>, Hudson Street Press, New York, 2013

[4] Johns Hopkins Medicine. "Physical fitness significantly improves survival, prevents heart attacks in people with stable coronary artery disease." *ScienceDaily*, 17 Nov. 2013. Web. 27 Nov. 2013.

[5] Nicholas Wade, "Your Body Is Younger Than You Think" <u>The New York Times</u>, August 2, 2005

[6] Bruce Alberts, Alexander Johnson, Julian Lewis, Martin Raff, Keith Roberts, and Peter Walter, <u>Molecular Biology of the Cell, 4th edition</u>, New York: Garland Science, 2002

[7] Michael Moss, "Safety of Beef Processing Method Is Questioned" <u>The New York Times</u>, December 30, 2009

[8] Renee Jacques, "These Disturbing Fast Food Truths Will Make You Reconsider Your Lunch" <u>The Huffington Post</u>, November 20, 2013

[9] Daniel Lieberman, <u>The Story of the Human Body: Evolution, Health, and Disease</u>, Pantheon Books, New York, 2013

[10] Daniel Lieberman, <u>The Story of the Human Body: Evolution, Health, and Disease</u>, Pantheon Books, New York, 2013

[11] Daniel Lieberman, <u>The Story of the Human Body: Evolution, Health, and Disease</u>, Pantheon Books, New York, 2013

[12] Robert H. Lustig, M.D., <u>Fat Chance: Beating the Odds Against Sugar, Processed Food, Obesity, and Disease</u>, Hudson Street Press, New York, 2013

[13] Donald Johanson, <u>Lucy: The Beginnings of Humankind</u>, Simon & Schuster, 1990

[14] Daniel Lieberman, <u>The Story of the Human Body: Evolution, Health, and Disease</u>, Pantheon Books, New York, 2013

[15] Robert H. Lustig, M.D., <u>Fat Chance: Beating the Odds Against Sugar, Processed Food, Obesity, and Disease</u>, Hudson Street Press, New York, 2013

[16] Robert H. Lustig, M.D., <u>Fat Chance: Beating the Odds Against Sugar, Processed Food, Obesity, and Disease</u>, Hudson Street Press, New York, 2013

[17] Publius Lawson, <u>The Invention of the Roller Flour Mill</u>, Nabu Press, 2014

[18] Pina LoGiudice ND, Lac and Peter Bongiorno ND, Lac, The Dr. Oz Show, "Why You Need Wheat Germ" http://www.doctoroz.com/videos/why-you-need-wheat-germ

[19] Michael Pollan, In Defense of Foods: An Eater's Manifesto, The Penguin Press, New York, 2008

[20] Robert H. Lustig, M.D., Fat Chance: Beating the Odds Against Sugar, Processed Food, Obesity, and Disease, Hudson Street Press, New York, 2013

[21] Harvard School of Public health, "Sugary Drinks", http://www.hsph.harvard.edu/nutritionsource/healthy-drinks/sugary-drinks/

[22] Marion Nestle and Malden Nesheim, Why Calories Count: From Science to Politics (California Studies in Food and Culture), University of California Press, London, England, 2012

[23] Mayo Clinic, "Artificial Sweeteners and Other Sugar Substitutes", http://www.mayoclinic.org/healthy-living/nutrition-and-healthy-eating/in-depth/artificial-sweeteners/art-20046936

[24] Emily Mann, Dr. Betty Martini, "7 Hidden Dangers of Artificial Sweeteners" http://www.rense.com/general96/artif.html

[25] Dr. Stanley Monteith, Dr. Russell Blaylock, Dr. Betty Martini, Aspartame: The Taste That Kills, Radio Library, 1999

[26] Harvard Health Publications, Harvard Medical School, http://www.health.harvard.edu/blog/artificial-sweeteners-sugar-free-but-at-what-cost-201207165030

[27] NYDailyNews.com, Overweight Americans who pick diet drinks consume more calories: study, January 17, 2014, http://www.nydailynews.com/life-style/health/obese-people-pick-diet-drinks-eat-food-study-article-1.1582996

[28] Mayo Clinic, Water: How much should you drink every day? http://www.mayoclinic.org/healthy-living/nutrition-and-healthy-eating/in-depth/water/art-20044256

[29] WebMD, "7 Wonders of Water" http://www.webmd.boots.com/diet/ss/slideshow-7-wonders-of-water

[30] Jim Thornton, "Is This the Most Dangerous Food for Men?" MensHealth.com May 19, 2009

[31] Sarah Terry, "Does Soy Protein Increase Estrogen Levels?" Livestrong.com August 16, 2013

[32] Gina Kolata, "Seeking Clues to Heart Disease in DNA of an Unlucky Family" The New York Times, May 12, 2013

[33] Molly McAdams, "Amino Acids in Soy Protein" Livestrong.com March 13, 2014

[34] Denise Minger, Death by Food Pyramid: How Shoddy Science, Sketchy Politics and Shady Special Interests Have Ruined Our Health, Primal Nutrition, Inc., 2014

[35] Gary Taubes, Why We Get Fat: And What to do About It, Anchor, 2011

[36] Nina Teicholz, "The Questionable Link Between Saturated Fat and Heart Disease" The Wall Street Journal, May 6, 2014

[37] Nina Teicholz, The Big Fat Surprise: Why Butter, Meat and Cheese Belong in a Healthy Diet, Simon & Schuster, New York, 2014

[38] American Heart Association, "Good vs. Bad Cholesterol" www.heart.org December 10, 2012

[39] Robert H. Lustig, M.D., <u>Fat Chance: Beating the Odds Against Sugar, Processed Food, Obesity, and Disease</u>, Hudson Street Press, New York, 2013

[40] Mayo Clinic, "Trans fat is double trouble for your heart health", May 6, 2011 http://www.mayoclinic.org/diseases-conditions/high-blood-cholesterol/in-depth/trans-fat/art-20046114

[41] Harvard School of Public Health, "Shining the Spotlight on Trans fats" http://www.hsph.harvard.edu/nutritionsource/transfats/

[42] American Heart Association, "Shaking the Salt Habit" www.heart.org March 5, 2014

[43] Sarah Albert, "How to Keep Your Veggies Vitamin Packed" www.webmd.com 2004

[44] Robert H. Lustig, M.D., <u>Fat Chance: Beating the Odds Against Sugar, Processed Food, Obesity, and Disease</u>, Hudson Street Press, New York, 2013

[45] Rubio-Tapia, PubMed.gov, "The prevalence of celiac disease in the United States" http://www.ncbi.nlm.nih.gov/pubmed/22850429

[46] Kenneth Chang, "Gluten-Free, Whether You Need It or Not" <u>The New York Times</u>, February 4, 2013

[47] Salynn Boyles, "Drinking Water May Speed Weight Loss" WebMD January 5, 2004

[48] Marion Nestle and Malden Nesheim, <u>Why Calories Count: From Science to Politics (California Studies in Food and Culture)</u>, University of California Press, London, England, 2012

[49] Paula Quinene, "Can Cardio Boost Metabolism?" Livestrong.com February 2, 2014

[50] Christian Thibaudeau, <u>The Black Book Of Training Secrets</u>, Francois Lepine; Enhanced Edition, 2007

[51] Mark Vella, <u>Anatomy for Strength and Fitness Training: An Illustrated Guide to Your Muscles in Action</u>, McGraw-Hill, 2006

[52] Wiki How to do anything, "How to Breathe Correctly While Bench Pressing" http://www.wikihow.com/Breathe-Correctly-While-Bench-Pressing

[53] Craig Smith, "When is Best Time for Protein Shakes?" Livestrong.com

http://www.livestrong.com/article/274794-when-is-best-time-for-protein-shakes, Aug 16, 2013

[54] Krista Scott-Dixon, PhD, "Maximize Your Workout With Protein & Nutrition Timing", The Diet Channel, http://www.thedietchannel.com/Protein-and-workout.htm, Oct 25, 2006

[55] Nicole Crawford, The Best Multivitamin Product, Livestrong.com http://www.livestrong.com/article/471295-the-best-multivitamin-product, 2011

[56] Andrea Cespedes, "Protein Bar Vs, Powder", Livestrong.com, http://www.livestrong.com/article/462471-protein-bar-vs-powder, June 2, 2014

[57] European Food Information Council, "Nutrient bioavailability – getting the most out of food." http://www.eufic.org/article/en/artid/Nutrient-bioavailability-food/ , May, 2010

References

[58] University of Maryland Medical Center, "Creatine" http://umm.edu/health/medical/altmed/supplement/creatine, April 9, 2011

[59] Murray Carpenter, <u>Caffeinated: How Our Daily Habit Helps, Hurts, and Hooks Us</u>, Hudson Street Press, New York, 2014

[60] Murray Carpenter, <u>Caffeinated: How Our Daily Habit Helps, Hurts, and Hooks Us</u>, Hudson Street Press, New York, 2014

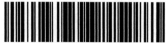

Made in the USA
Lexington, KY
18 June 2015